Praise for
Be Young and B

Everyone ages. But few people have the idea and plan as to how to deal with it. This book gives you very important insight and real solutions you would need to know to respond to the challenge of aging of our body, mind and spirit!

—YUE-SAI KAN, MEDIA ICON, SUCCESSFUL ENTREPRENEUR, BEST SELLING AUTHOR

As East moves closer to the West, we are expanding out appreciation of the millennia of knowledge, both practical and spiritual, that has now been delivered to us. The delivery of this combined approach to a healthier and happier life comes by way of this new book by my dear friends and colleague. This book is a must read for anyone wanting a brighter and healthier future life. Read it, absorb it, use it, and share in the knowledge with all those that you care for.

—DR. MARK GORDON, MEDICAL DIRECTOR, MILLENNIUM HEALTH CENTERS

A unique blend of modern medical perspectives, traditional medical knowledge and philosophy . . . diligently researched and articulately presented.

—DR. HANS KIERSTEAD, CO-DIRECTOR, SUE AND BILL GROSS STEM CELL RESEARCH CENTER, UNIVERSITY OF CALIFORNIA, IRVINE.

The best of all healing worlds—modern Western medicine blended with centuries-old Oriental wisdom. This book deserves to be on every health-seeker's bookshelf. I thoroughly enjoyed it!

—ANN LOUISE GITTLEMAN,
AUTHOR OF *THE FAT FLUSH PLAN*

This book is so full of so much valuable information. Drs. Tzu and Wu have put together arguably one of the most complete compendiums to optimal health and wellbeing.

—DR. MARK BERMAN, PRESIDENT OF THE AMERICAN
ACADEMY OF COSMETIC SURGERY

When it comes to living a long life, it is the quality of those years that counts, not the quantity. Every week more books on longevity and healthy aging are appearing on store shelves, but I have seen few as comprehensive and innovative as *Be Young and Beyond*. Blended with the latest research, *Be Young and Beyond* gives you a complete, 360-degree roadmap to synergistically create a more youthful, vibrant, abundant and longer life. Its plan may just save your life—or the life of someone you love. This is a must read!

—DR. LEIGH ERIN CONNEALY, MD,
MEDICAL DIRECTOR, CENTER FOR NEW MEDICINE

As an Exercise Physiologist for over 40 years and a teacher of aging and exercise, I found that *Be Young and Beyond* by Dr. Taichi Tzu and Dr. Ping Wu is most comprehensive approach I've read to date. It definitely has become a complete "How To" be young and functional. They have tapped into the real science of staying ageless. Taichi and Ping are living examples of their work.

—GORDON DUFFY, MFS, CSCS CHEK, PRESIDENT, DUFFY FITNESS INSTITUTE, AUTHOR OF *FORGET EVERYTHING YOU EVER HEARD ABOUT EXERCISE*

This book provides a distinctive view of holistic health and is well worth a careful reading.

—DR. DAVID HEBER, DIRECTOR, UCLA CENTER FOR HUMAN NUTRITION

Congratulations to Dr. Li and Dr. Wu for a most insightful book. They truly understand that whatever comes into or affects our bodies needs to be optimal and precise and not excessive.

—DR. DAVID DITSWORTH, MEDICAL DIRECTOR, THE BACK INSTITUTE, BEVERLY HILLS

I'm so happy to see this unique and fascinating work, demonstrating an artful combination of science and Taoism, not only in the authors' years of cultivation on themselves, but also finally in print to benefit all.

—HE NANJIE, GRAND TAICHI MASTER AND TAOIST

BE YOUNG AND BEYOND

A LIFELONG JOURNEY TO VIBRANT HEALTH & LONGEVITY

Taichi Tzu, Ph.D., and
Ping Wu, M.D., Ph.D.

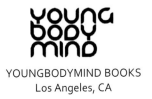

YOUNGBODYMIND BOOKS
Los Angeles, CA

Published in the United States by: YoungBodyMind Books,
a division of YoungBodyMind LLC
Los Angeles, The United States of America

ISBN 978–09831655–6–9

Library of Congress Control Number: 2010941505

Cover and text design: Gary A. Rosenberg
Editor: Kathleen Barnes

This book is not intended to replace medical advice or to be a substitute for a physician. We advise the reader to consult with a physician before beginning any program in this book. The authors disclaim any liability, personal or otherwise, resulting from the procedures in this book.

Contents

*Dedicated to a healthier and
more spiritually developed mankind*

Acknowledgements

A special thanks to the thousands of patients who have been on this journey with us in the quest for the optimal ways towards vibrant health and longevity.

Our gratitude also goes to our friends and some of the most respected doctors and scientists in the fields anti-aging and regenerative medicine who have so generously exchanged ideas with us: Dr. Mark Gordon, Dr. Mark Berman, Dr. Gordon Duffy, Dr. Paul McAndrews, Dr. Karlis Ullis, Dr. David Ditsworth, Dr. Larry Milam, Dr. Leigh Erin Connealy, Dr. Fouad Ghaly, Dr. Karen Sun, Dr. Sharon McQuillan, Dr. Jim Bell, Dr. James Privitera, Dr. Nicholai Tankovich, Dr. Mingzhe Chen, Dr. Alex Khrazi, Dr. David Howe, Dr. Hans Kierstead, Dr. Habib Torfi, Dr. Roger Miesfeld.

Our thanks to our friends and fellow doctors and scientists in the root of Tradition Chinese Medicine, Dr. Liu Fenjun, Professor Cheng Xinong, Dr. Changshan Xin.

A special thanks to our dear friends Yue-Sai Kan, R.J. Brandes and Elizabeth Segerstrom for their ideas and encouragement.

We are deeply indebted to our Taoist teacher, Grand Tai-Chi Master Nanjie Ho and the many mystic teachers of Taoism and Buddhism who live anonymously deep inside of the sacred mountains of China away from all the worldly materialism.

We are thankful for the unfailing support from our family, Justin Li, Jason Li, Wang Xin, Bao Yiaxian, Li Sitian, and Wu Shouxin.

We give special thanks to the editorial help provided by Kathleen Barnes of Take Charge Books for her contribution to our completion of the book.

Preface

This book is about PingLongevity™, a complete program to help you live a more youthful, vibrant and longer life. The goal is to age at half the rate of those who live a conventional lifestyle and to dramatically increase your lifespan while looking and feeling decades younger than others in the same age group.

You may ask, "Why another program?"

Every day renowned gurus, doctors, scientists and drug companies flood the market with new diet plans, weight loss schemes, magic exercises, dietary supplements and new drugs, all promising effective results.

Do these plans work? Why is there so much more obesity, diabetes, cancer and other degenerative diseases today? You may have tried these methods—or similar ones—one after the other. You may wonder why they don't work as claimed. You may wonder why even the promoters frequently fail to show personal results that validate their product claims.

We have found that vibrant health is achievable only through a complete approach. Our decades of research and clinical applications on ourselves and many thousands of patients have made it clear that you cannot expect to use a one-pill-fix-all method. In many cases, experts, although excellent in their own fields, give too much credit to a particular diet, exercise, pill, nutrient or method. The one-pill-fix-all approach plays well to consumer psychology in that we all want an easy fix-it-all elixir! The fact is that these miracle approaches rarely achieve the expected results.

Our work is not another fashionable "free lunch" on longevity—hot for a couple of years, only to be proven ineffective. What we present is a true journey to vibrant health. PingLongevity™ is different, in the following aspects:

- It is a complete way of life, only through which you can achieve long-lasting vibrant health and longevity. There is no short cut.

- It combines thousands of years of Taoist longevity, based on the I-Ching energy cycle, five elements, yin-yang, Taoist alchemy and extensive scientific research. It peels to the very core and explains the things that really make a difference.

- It works not only on the physical, but also the energy level of our bodies. It deals with body, mind and spirit.

- It shows you the correct ways of diet, caloric restriction, hormone balance and exercise.

- It surveys up-to-date biomedical and medical advances in the anti-aging field.

This book could have been several volumes, due to the breadth of the subjects covered. However, we attempted to give you a complete program all in one book in as concise a form as possible because missing even one piece of the full PingLongevity™ puzzle would not give you total health.

Why the name PingLongevity™? It comes from the Chinese word "Ping," meaning peace, health and luck. The program is an advancement from our previous books, *PingLongevity,* and *Asian Longevity Secrets,* published nearly 10 years ago.

We look at the book as a give-back to the society where we have been so fortunate to build our lives, careers, knowledge and spirituality. It's our desire to contribute to the happiness and vibrant health of millions of people. This book is dedicated to a healthier and more spiritually developed mankind.

Taichi Tzu, Ph.D.
Ping Wu, M.D, Ph.D.

CHAPTER 1

PingLongevity™ Defined

Do you really want a long and healthy life? We often hear friends say that they don't want to live to an extreme old age. Instead, they just want to be healthy when they live.

Yes, we agree. But isn't that our real purpose, to extend a vital and productive life? If you are 50, but feel, function and look like you are in your late 20s, or at 70 but look and feel like you are 40, isn't that nice? All of us would love it.

Additionally, almost all degenerative diseases such as cancer, heart disease, Type 2 diabetes, Alzheimer's and Parkinson's are associated with aging. Many experts now think aging is itself the root cause of many of degenerative diseases. From this point of view, a goal of longevity is consistent with living a healthy, youthful and vibrant life. If you can delay aging, you can also delay or prevent these diseases.

PingLongevity™ is a way of life that allows you to age at a half the rate as others, maximizing your productive lifespan. Our goal is to maintain a youthful, healthy and vibrant life for 120 years or more.

1.1   YOUNG AND VIBRANT FOR 120 YEARS

Yes, it's possible. However, there are no magic pills for immortality. A real science of regeneration, anti-aging, longevity and life extension is a complex process that requires a complete approach. That is why history has recorded so many magic pills, shots and drugs that never worked!

Think of the well-known experts in diet, nutrition, endocrinology, Ayurvedic medicine, Chinese medicine and conventional medicine. Though they may be at the top of their own fields, few could demonstrate any biological proof they have slowed or stopped the aging process.

The complexity of human health and longevity is similar to the ancient Chinese story of blind men attempting to describe an elephant, each of them touching only one part of the whole. Thus, each man comes up with a different viewpoint: the trunk method, the tusk method, the ear method, the tail method, the leg method and so on. Although they are all experts of their own "fields," they unfortunately cannot describe the elephant as the whole.

The fact is that a million things can be proven beneficial to human health in one way or another. There are hundreds of thousands of herbs, fruits, and vegetables in nature, all of which can be proven to have some health benefit, such as reducing the risk of cancer. But can we take them all? Is the effect too insignificant to be really practically useful?

Only in recent years have some scientific and medical authorities begun to accept the following conditions as diseases:

- **Sub-health:** Defined by the World Health Organization as a state between health and medically defined "disease," sub-health occurs when no definable disease is present after conventional medical testing, but the person experiences all kinds of discomfort and pain. These should be considered the "new killer" or "chronic and silent diseases." Many such maladies have been labeled "syndromes," which means there is a wide array of symptoms, but conventional medicine has not yet devised an effective treatment.

  Consider the following: chronic fatigue, insomnia, forgetfulness, somnolence, heavy dreaming, dizziness, distention, mental fatigue, cumbersome limbs, shoulder and back soreness, lack of concentration, proneness to flu and cold, poor appetite, dizziness, blurred vision, anxiety and depression, agitation, shortness of breath, restlessness, irregular menses, poor sexual performance, palpitations and weight gain. These are all symptoms of sub-health.

- **Silent inflammation:** Introduced by leading anti-aging doctors, silent inflammation is the underlying cause of all age-related degenerative diseases. It takes years of such silent inflammation before serious diseases become apparent.

- **Loss of tissue function:** Many organs do not test positive for disease until a large percentage of tissues lose their ability to function. For example, the term "chronic kidney disease" (CKD) was not a standard medical definition until 2002. In standard medical tests BUN (blood urea nitrogen) and creatinine, indicators of chronic kidney disease may not change beyond the "normal range" until 60% of total kidney function is lost and the disease is far progressed.

- **Aging:** Now accepted as a disease by many leading experts, aging is certainly a risk factor of many degenerative diseases such as diabetes, heart disease, Alzheimer's, Parkinson's and obesity. The job of new medicine is to delay aging, thus reduce disease. The biological aging process can be slowed by early detection of changing biomarkers of aging such as hormone imbalance, nutrition imbalance, toxicity and autoimmune disorders plus treating the fundamental causes using natural methods of integrative medicine.

PingLongevity™ is a scientific way of life that combines the best of integrative medicine, anti-aging medicine, regenerative medicine, traditional Chinese medicine, Taoist alchemy and many new treatments and innovations. The focus is on early detection and prevention of chronic and often silent conditions before they evolve into sub-health problems and diseases.

The renowned Traditional Chinese Medicine (TCM) doctor, Bian Que, said some 3,000 years ago:

"Top doctors prevent diseases before they manifest, middle level doctors heal sub-health and bottom level doctors treat diseases."

From our viewpoint, illness is due to long-term silent disease and sub-health as a result of the aging process and unhealthy lifestyle. These conditions become chronic and evolve into disease conditions because of a lack of early detection and an unhealthy lifestyle. Therefore, PingLongevity™ focuses on preventing illness before it can manifest.

Is this possible? Yes, entirely so.

In this section, we give you an outline of the entire Ping-Longevity™ program. There is no free lunch here. The more you're able to follow this way of life, the more you'll benefit from a longer and more vital life.

1.1.1   You Are What You Eat

For the sake of simplicity, let us use an analogy of our automobiles. We feed our cars with gasoline. Our cars burn gasoline with the help of oxygen and create energy to drive. But no engine is 100% efficient. It produces byproducts that oxidize the engine. Over time, the engine becomes old and needs replacement. So some of us like to use cleaner gas to help our cars stay cleaner and last longer.

Very similarly, we humans burn glucose or sugar derived from foods, mixed with oxygen breathed in from the lungs to produce energy for the cells in our bodies. Burning glucose also oxidizes and ages our bodies. Therefore, we must use the cleanest and most nutrition-rich, calorie-efficient foods.

What you eat can make a world of difference in your entire health and longevity. Think about what might happen if you adopt a daily breakfast plan that is vastly superior to what most others eat:

- 40% fewer calories;

- 86% less saturated fat;

- 650% more omega-3 fatty acid;

- 99% less cholesterol

- 5000 oxygen radical absorbance capacity (ORAC) as compared with almost none;

- Loads of vitamins and minerals from super green vegetables as compared with none;

- Complete raw with full loads of natural digestive enzymes as compared with cooked zero-enzyme foods.

What if you do this day in and day out for years? You'll definitely beat the odds in favor of super health and longevity. We'll discuss the PingLongevity™ Diet in Chapter 2.

1.1.2   The Only Scientifically Proven Way of Extending Maximum Life Span

Again let's look at cars. A car can run about 150,000 miles in its lifetime. If you drive 30,000 miles a year, the car can last 5 years. But if you only drive 10,000 miles a year, it'll last 15 years. So the car's lifespan depends on the rate at which we use it. This applies to humans too. Theoretically, a human can live 120 years healthy and disease-free. But our lifespan also depends on our rate of living. This is the so-called metabolic rate. If we can make our metabolism so efficient, say, as to live the same lifestyle but consuming only one half of the calories that those activities usually require, we can cut our rate of aging by half. This has been scientifically proven to be possible.

Studies on rats conducted by Dr. Roy Walford at the UCLA School of Medicine in 1986 also demonstrated the dramatic extension of lifespan. Rats have a maximum lifespan of around 35 months, equivalent to a human's 120 years. Every 10 months of a rat's lifetime is equivalent to about 34 human years. Experiments have shown that a 50% caloric restriction delays aging by 18 months in rats, equivalent to about 60 years in a human.

Further studies on monkeys led by Prof. Weindruch of University of Wisconsin-Madison and humans in the Biosphere Project (published in *Annals of Academy of Sciences*) further proved the science of caloric restriction without malnutrition.

We can tune our bodies, making them dramatically more fuel-efficient engines than people not practicing the caloric restriction method. You'll learn about PingLongevity™ Caloric Restriction in Chapter 3.

1.1.3   Most People Exercise Wrong

Your body is like a machine. If you use it too much, it wears and tears. It is like anything: It gets old. On the other hand, if you don't use it, it loses functionality. This, of course, includes your entire body: heart, lung, eyes, ears, arms, legs, midsection, neck, brain, etc.

When one 70-year-old patient told us that she bought a sandal hook so that she wouldn't have to bend over to put her shoes on, we cautioned her that, even if it's hard to bend down, if she does not try it, she'll gradually lose that capability completely, once for all.

The real science of exercise is to maintain all the necessary body functionality while creating minimum wear and tear!

Many of you go to the gym "to burn more calories." This is a wrong objective. Why? Suppose we set a goal for our car to burn at least 20 gallons of gas a week even if we don't need that much for our weekly commute. We just drive around mindlessly for the purpose of burning more gas. Are we out of our minds?

The correct purpose of exercise is for cardiovascular and respiratory capacity, for muscle and bone strength and for flexibility. There is also a need for exercising the brain and the eyes.

Exercise may also be necessary to help rehabilitate us after an injury or surgery. But we must engage in intelligent exercise and not create overuse. We must do it to the point where the body keeps its functionality with minimum wear and tear. To learn more about this, go to Chapter 4 for PingLongevity™ Exercise.

1.1.4   Don't Block Your Energy Channels

It's quite simple to convince yourself of the existence of energy channels or meridians and energy centers or acupuncture points in your body. Just sit still, close your eyes, and rest your hands with palms facing up. Send your thoughts to your hands. Pretty soon, you'll feel warmth in your hands. This simple test shows that your mind can move your blood and chi (energy). Over time, most of us develop blockages in energy channels. When we are energetically out of balance, we get sick and we age

Chapter 5 will discuss the basis of PingLongevity™ Energy Balance, which tells us how to balance our body meridians using Traditional Chinese Medicine (TCM) methods and Taoist chi-gong.

1.1.5   Stress Can Age You Fast!

We've all inherited the ability of fight or flight from our ancestors. When you run into a tiger in a forest, your body suddenly enters into an emergency state, widely opening all fight or flight functions, pumping sugar (energy) into the muscles and shutting down all non-fighting related functions, such as digestion. Modern stress turns our bodies into chronic fight and flight machines that never turn off. That's the source of most of our diseases and aging.

Stress, greed and craving unnecessary emotional stimulation leak your precious spiritual energy. In Chapter 6, we talk about PingLongevity™ Spirit for preventing such leaks.

1.1.6   Hormones and Aging

You may easily imagine what would happen if your car's brakes fail. What if the airbag system fails? Then what if the fuel injection controls, AC and timing system are all out of sync?

Hormones, also known as the endocrine system, are your body's control system. As you age, most of your hormones decline and they become unbalanced. When they become unbalanced, diseases such as cancer, heart disease, obesity and osteoporosis arise. Therefore, maintaining a good hormonal level and keeping hormones in balance is critically important to your well-being. However, hormone balance is a hugely complex science. Just like tuning your car is a complex process, hormones, if not tuned properly, can expose the body to many side effects. Thus, the goal is to maintain a youthful hormone level and balance while doing it correctly so that to avoid all the potential risk. PingLongevity™ Hormone is the main focus of Chapter 7.

1.1.7   Look and Act Young

Psychologically accepting aging makes you old. Are you:

- Afraid of tinkering with the new generation of electronic gadgets?

- Unable to perform on the Internet or e-mail?

- Paying little attention to the fashions of the younger generation?

- Only interested in decades-old music?

- Giving up the fight against wrinkles and accepting your growing belly or blossoming hips?

- Only socializing with people your age or older?

The world continues to move forward. If you don't keep up, you get old. When you accept being old, your body, mind and spirit fall behind, too.

Chapter 8, PingLongevity™ Look talks about natural ways of keeping a younger look and a youthful outlook on life.

1.1.8   You May Still Need Intervention

There are two ways of slowing the aging process: through lifestyle and by intervention.

The best way is to use lifestyle to keep yourself young and healthy naturally for as long as possible. Intervention should only be used as a last resort.

Chapters 2–8 will give you the fundamental lifestyle changes you'll need to make to extend your youthful and vibrant health for as long as possible. Unlike new technologies that always advance, this lifestyle advice never changes because it is based on the physiological definitions of the human body and mind.

Sooner or later you may still need intervention with new bio-medical technologies and treatment methods, including bio-identical hormone replacement, stem cell therapy or gene therapy. This is the subject of Chapter 9.

1.1.9 Life as Energy

Can man live without food? Can man be immortal? What happens after we die? These are some fundamental questions related to longevity. Science has only started to scratch the surface of these questions.

Chapter 10 is an attempt to provide a framework for a hypothesis to shed some light on energy and life.

1.2 WHAT HAPPENS WHEN WE AGE?

In this section, we discuss a few major aspects of aging. Don't get depressed or discouraged by the grim aspects of aging. All the unpleasantness can be delayed and even prevented and reversed entirely as you follow the PingLongevity™ plan outlined in this book.

1.2.1 The Decline of Biomarkers of Aging

Medically, true biomarkers of aging have to reflect a universal species characteristic, somewhat independent of environment, geography and lifestyle. For example, blood cholesterol is not a good marker because even though for most of the time, cholesterol goes up with age, in some societies, it does not. Similarly, driving without a safety belt is not a biomarker of aging, even if it might be a biomarker of early mortality.

The following biomarkers, showing changes between ages 20 to 60, are true measures of functional age accepted by scientists. We'll discuss their measurement further in Section 1.4.

- Skin elasticity reduced by 15-fold;

- Lung vital capacity (VC), measured by the amount of air that can be taken in and breathed out in one very deep breath, declines about 40%. The VO2 Max, maximum consumption rate of oxygen during strenuous exercise such as walking on jogging on a tread-mill, declines about 25%, thus lessening the ability to play intense sports.

- Hearing threshold (at 8000 Hz) requires the sound to be 8 times louder as we age;

- Static balance, the ability to stand on one foot with closed eyes, decreases 6-fold;

- Reaction time (falling ruler test score) deteriorates by 60%;

- Visual accommodation, ability to read close up, deteriorates by 8.7-fold;

- Systolic blood pressure increases by 20%;

- Creatinine clearance, a measure of kidney function, declines by 20%;

- Insulin sensitivity (measured by glucose tolerance test), a meas-ure of the sensitivity of your insulin production to glucose intake, deteriorates by 19%;

- Autoantibodies, a measure of autoimmune diseases, increase by 5-fold.

In the next few sub-sections, we talk about other indicators of aging, not necessarily scientifically classified as true biomarkers.

1.2.2 The Decline of Hormonal Control System

Hormones are the controls in your body. Hormones tend to change both in levels and their interrelationship as we age:

- Growth hormone decreases dramatically causing the so-called *somatopause,* causing lost muscle, sagging skin, obesity, etc.;

- Thyroid gland enters into *thyropause* with age, especially in women. Fully 25% of postmenopausal women have either clinical or subclinical hypothyroidism, causing symptoms such as depression, memory loss, cognitive impairment and a variety of neuromuscular complaints.

- Adrenal glands decline with age, causing the so-called *adrenopause,* or *adrenal fatigue,* correlating to a decline of immune response and increase of diabetes, atherosclerosis, dementia, obesity and osteoporosis.

- Metabolic Syndrome or Syndrome X becomes prevalent. Each time we eat, insulin is released into the bloodstream. This vital hormone, secreted by the pancreas, encourages our tissues—our muscles in particular—to gobble up the glucose surging through the bloodstream after we eat a meal. As we age, the body's response to insulin becomes less sensitive causing a high level of blood sugar lingering in the blood for many hours, which is a fundamental cause of Type 2 diabetes and increased cholesterol, triglycerides and blood pressure.

- Women usually begin *menopause* in their late 40s and *perimenopause* as early as their mid 30s. Between the ages of 35 and 55, women experience significant hormonal changes, causing various symptoms and diseases such as heart disease, osteoporosis, diabetes, obesity and endometrial and breast cancer.

- Men begin *andropause* in their late 40s or as early as their mid 30s with a gradual change in hormone levels, leading to many symptoms and degenerative diseases such as impotence, cardiovascular diseases, depression, metabolic syndrome and prostate cancer.

1.2.3 Accumulated Wear and Tear with Lost Functionality

Just like any object—furniture, car, machine, tool—our bodies get worn out as we age:

- Joints become less functional due to arthritis (wearing and tearing of bones);

- Cartilage and discs become worn out, eliminating natural joint cushions and causing bones to rub together;

- Skin bears sun damage, scars, wrinkles and all the signs of wear and tear;

- Muscles carry lifelong injuries such as pulls, tears and cuts;

- Eardrums become damaged due to lifelong exposure to loud sounds;

- Organ tissues become scarred due to lifelong viral attack;

- Cells grow older, losing their regenerative and repair capabilities;

- Many bodily functions and normal movement are lost due to inactivity (e.g., flexibility, especially in the spine).

1.2.4   Changes in the Way We Look

As we age, our appearance begins to change due to these underlying causes:

- Postural changes related to bone structure (osteoporosis, damage and drying of soft bones such as cartilage and discs, arthritis):
  - Rigid movement;
  - Shortened height;
  - Curved spine;

- Fat redistribution:
  - Fat disappears from the face and neck causing skin sagging with a tired and hollow look, mimicking a skeleton head;
  - Fat accumulates in the mid-section, belly in men and hips and upper legs in women;

- Hair redistribution, especially for men:
  - Receding hair at temples;
  - Balding, which may be more genetic than a product of aging;

- ○ Overall thinning hair in the head, even without balding, most men at middle age have lost about 50% of their hair density;

- ○ Heavier hair at the tips of eyebrows, nose, nipples, chest;

- Reduced skin elasticity:
  - ○ Uneven thickness of skin—thinning on the face, neck, hands and thickening in mid sections;
  - ○ Drying and wrinkling of skin;

- Weight change:
  - ○ Weight increases to about age 60, then begins to fall as we grow older due mostly to loss of lean tissue, muscle mass, water and bone.

1.2.5　The Lost Mental Capacity

Brain function is also reduced as we age. About 35% of people develop Alzheimer's disease by age 75 and 50% develop it by age 85.

1.2.6　The Impact of the Advancement of Mankind

This is, in the strictest sense, not so much related to our physiology and the biochemistry of aging. However, as we grow older, our societies continue to advance, bringing dramatic changes around us. Some changes will positively impact our aging, while others will be negative.

Advances in medical technology and food preservation, storage, processing and transportation have dramatically increased lifespan of mankind, especially reflected in a reduced mortality rate.

However, there are also many side effects of so-called "advances" that are causing an increased occurrence of degenerative diseases, as well as the obesity epidemic:

- The processed food industry has denatured our food supply, with foods full of preservatives, deprived of natural digestive enzymes and with little nutritional value;

- The new genetically-engineered crops and hormone-fed animals have introduced new health challenges, including increased prevalence of allergies, toxicity, hormone imbalance and cancer-causing substances;

- Modern day chronic stress focused on materialism has dramatically caused imbalance of our hormonal systems;

- Chemicals in detergents, household cleaners, air, water, utensils and even furniture and clothing has increased our exposure to toxins and cancer-causing agents;

- Waves of electrical transmissions, radio frequency communication and radiation have a dramatic impact on our bodies' electromagnetic systems.

1.3 THEORIES OF AGING

There are actually living things that age very slowly, such as sharks, sea turtles and whales. Rockfish, the ones we eat at our dinner table, are usually over 100 years old. Nobody really knows why.

There are more than 25 modern and a great many more ancient theories on aging. It's impossible for us to talk about them all. But let's mention a few of them.

1.3.1   Procreation Theory

The Disposable Soma theory is based on a hypothesis that the purpose of our bodies and lives is for procreation only. Thus after procreation, life is no longer necessary. Evolution has selected the species that maximize procreation of offspring at the expense of longer life.

1.3.2   Wear and Tear Hypothesis

Another theory is based on the Wear and Tear hypothesis. Animals including ourselves, get old, just like cars do, and eventually we simply break down and are unable to function anymore. Elephants die because they wear down their teeth so much that they can no longer eat properly.

1.3.3   Rate of Living Hypothesis

Another theory uses a Rate of Living hypothesis. It states that there is a metabolic "bank account." We have a finite amount of total fuel or calories throughout life. The quicker we consume that total, the faster we die.

1.3.4   Oxidative Stress Theory

There is also the Oxidative Stress theory. You often hear about free radicals and antioxidants in dietary supplement ads. This theory says that as we metabolize glucose as fuel, the free oxygen radicals combine with proteins, etc., to form damaged cells. As time goes by, these damaged cells accumulate, just as rust inside a car engine accumulates over time. Since our bodies burn fuel (glucose) with the help of oxygen breathed in through the lungs and carried by blood, we have a mechanism similar to an automobile engine burning gasoline with the help of air (or oxygen). No body system or car engine is 100% efficient, so byproducts are created over time. Oxides are the biggest byproduct, creating rust in the inner parts of a car's engine. Oxides also 'rust' the cells of our bodies.

1.4   MEASURING AND MONITORING AGING AND HEALTH

For an effective measurement system, we must understand not only what to measure, but also recognize the optimal targets. There is an enormous amount of misinformation and ignorance on the subject of optimal targets. Only when we understand the optimal targets can we start to talk about how we can move our health towards the optimal. This section will talk about the framework of Ping-Longevity™ Test.

1.4.1   What Is Your Ideal or Optimal Health Target?

A car needs to be tuned up periodically. Tune up parameters are perfectly specified. Some of us take annual physicals, if we have that luxury. When you undergo medical testing, the doctors compare your results to the normal range, which is based on the statistical range of thousands of people. Usually that range is so wide that unless there are major problems, your results are negative. Then all we get from the doctor is a big stamp of "normal" without doing any preventative maintenance.

For example, the medical normal range of testosterone for an adult male is 270–1070 ng/dL. If a man has a level of 500 ng/dL, is he normal, too low, or too high? The answer may be any of the three choices depending on the situation. You may have had testosterone levels of 1000 when you were 20 years old, young and vibrant. Now your test result of 500 is 50% reduction from your peak. You're definitely in pretty severe hormone decline and imbalance. You'll run the risk of many degenerative diseases. On the other hand, you may have your level at 600 when you're young and vibrant. Now at 500, with a 15% decline, you may still be just fine.

We also have more progressive doctors who artificially set the "normal" bar higher. For example, we often hear famous anti-aging doctors say that even though the normal range of growth hormone (measured as IGF-1) is 109–284 ng/mL, we all should have a level of 300 ng/mL, above the maximum "normal" range to function well. This can be very risky without understanding what is optimal to a specific individual.

In the PingLongevity™ Test, we believe that your optimal or ideal measurement target should be benchmarked to you as an individual, not the general population. If you were healthy when you were young, your optimal benchmark is your levels at the ages of 18 to 22.

You should try to record every parameter of your health when you are as close to your early 20s as possible, provided that you're healthy at that age, so you have an optimal benchmark for later in life.

Most of us don't have the fortune to have recorded the optimal benchmark when we were young because there was simply no one to tell us so and perhaps many of the benchmarks were not even known at that time. Don't panic! A good doctor will not only look at the lab normal range, but also use qualitative tests and other analytical means to detect symptoms of imbalance. Intervention methods can also be used in small increments to make sure you don't surpass the maximum levels.

1.4.2 Biological Age versus Chronological Age

You have probably heard about biological age or real age. You may wonder what that means. Some people look and function much younger than their chronological or calendar age. Fundamentally, they age more slowly. We are talking about aging of cells, organs, functions, etc. Therefore, theoretically, there is a biological age and it is very possible to have a biological age younger than your chronological age. On the other hand, there are people who are biologically older than their chronological age.

Many doctors, institutions and gurus will tell you they can measure your biological age. Often they do some measurements and tell you that you're much older or much younger than your age. They do this based on statistical averages. For example, some leading doctors give you a biological age based on a bone density DEXA scan. On average, bone density ranges from 1 to 4. Based on some statistics, they draw a line to associate each measurement with an age, for example, a "1" for a healthy 20- to 30-year-old, and perhaps a "4" for a 70-year-old. You may be a 31-year-old, get a #3 measurement, so you'll be told your biological age is 55.

These are actually only to reference the average population, rather than to predict your own biological age or real age. To illustrate the issue, let's study the following case:

"At 29, I wanted to do an early benchmark of my hormone levels, when I was still at my peak health and vitality. When my growth hormone results (IGF-1) came back, my level was 195 ng/mL. The report from this leading anti-aging organization said my result corresponded to the levels expected in a 75-year-old, and that I should seek hormone replacement to increase the level to 300. I was so discouraged. In consulting with Dr. Ping, she told me I'm young, perfectly healthy and have no symptoms of any hormone imbalance or deficiency, so I may personally be genetically optimal with a lower level than what the test lab thinks I should have. Now, 15 years later, I'm still very healthy and through a healthy lifestyle, I am able to keep my hormone levels very close to where I was in my late 20s."

—Eric, Los Angeles

In Eric's case, if a doctor decided it was necessary to raise his IGF-1 level towards a "normal" 300 ng/mL, he may have some serious problems due to severe hormone imbalance.

Frank, a patient, came to the PingClinic one day. Here's his dialogue with Dr. Ping:

"I just had a biomarker test given by an anti-aging doctor. He told me I am functionally ten years older than my age. He said I needed to use growth hormones."

"How did you do in the categories he tested?" asked Dr. Ping.

"Not well in what is called the forced vital capacity test. The doctor explained that it measures lung function, the amount of air that can be inhaled and exhaled rapidly in one very deep breath. Although I'm 45, I scored a functional age of 60-plus. I also did poorly in a growth hormone test, IGF-1, again about that of a 60-year-old. I thought I was healthier than most people my age. But now I am depressed."

"How was your lung function when you were young?"

"I don't know. I was a 100-meter medalist in high school and college. But I wasn't good at longer ranges, such as 800 meters or 1500 meters. I got tired and out of breath easily."

"So your lung capacity wasn't that high when you were young. Most probably the same test then would have given similar results," said Dr. Ping.

"You think so?"

"Yes, each one of us is different. We were born to be strong in certain areas and weak in others. This does not mean that we were born to be functionally old. Tests, like the ones you have recently undergone, use statistical averages as their reference range. For example, if your test results fall into a range among average Americans in your age group, you are considered medically normal. You may have a lower blood pressure of 90/65 compared with your age group, but if you have been at this level all your life and you are healthy, you are fine. You must compare yourself today with your own historical test results. Look for the trend. If the trend takes a downturn at a rate faster than the average, you are aging faster. Doctors can only conclude that you are somewhat within or out of the normal range. But telling your functional age is another matter. I think you may find yourself in the normal functional age for the vital capacity test if you compare the results to your own history as a youth."

"What about the tests where I did well?"

"What was your BMI, the body-mass index?"

"About 22. For six feet, 190 pounds, it's perfect, according to the Centers for Disease Control and Prevention standard. I am proud of myself. You know, 61% of Americans are considered overweight," said Frank.

"Remember what I said: Compare yourself with yourself, not with the average. What was your weight at age 20?" asked Dr. Ping, wanting to drive the concept home so Frank could get a correct perception of his health.

"I was about 155 pounds," he said. He thought it over and added, "You think maybe I am a little overweight compared to my own standard? True, I'm okay compared with the average. But since I was thinner than average genetically, I need to be thinner than the average BMI."

"Exactly. A person's ideal weight is when he is at his peak energy, which is around 18 to 22 years old. As we age, we tend to put on additional weight unnecessarily. We burn our engines, not for useful work, but to make useless fat. Since the engine can only run a certain number of miles, we accelerate aging unnecessarily. Ideally, if you want to keep your functional youth, maintain your ideal weight throughout life," concluded Dr. Ping.

The point here is that due to a large variation of each individual's genetic composition, your biological age can only be compared with yourself. We may function as healthy, as normal and young even if our parameters come from the statistics derived from a large number of people. Therefore, unless you have been tracking your health parameters consistently over the years, it's difficult to precisely estimate your biological age. You may only be qualitatively evaluated as much younger, much older, about the same, etc.

Our approach is different. We don't believe functional age can be accurately estimated. Few of us tracked our biomarkers when we were 20 years old, so there is little to compare. After all, the purpose is to understand if we are changing rapidly and to figure out ways to slow down or reverse the changes. Therefore, we think testing is for identification of issues and trends, rather than estimating biological age.

1.4.3   Misconception of Youthfulness

Many people brag about how they were once prone to colds when they were young, but now they seldom get sick. Is this an indication of youthfulness? Maybe not. Think about young people. Children are usually very susceptible to colds and when they get colds, they may also have severe symptoms. When you're bragging about never getting minor illnesses, you might want to know why your immune system is so insensitive to viruses, bacteria, etc. That's why some people frequently get sick throughout their lives, but live very long without terminal diseases. On the other hand, some people who are considered super healthy, suddenly find themselves developing a serious illness.

Some guys never developed large defined muscles when they were young, partly because they genetically belong to a different type and partly due to their lack of desire to get into sports. Many healthy young people belong in this category. However, we often hear about men who suddenly show off how muscular they have become when they are into their 50s. They become gym rats and take lots of proteins, hormone stimulators and even hormones.

Does this necessarily indicate a younger physiology than when they were young? Definitely not. When you deviate from your natural genetic disposition, you risk the danger of major imbalance and disease. Be content with who you are.

The point here is that there are many misconceptions about what we are looking for. PingLongevity™ is a way of life to keep you young, compared to your own body's physiology, for as long as possible. However, if you were not an athlete, an "often-get-a colder" and a thin guy in your youth, so be it. It's not what we are concerned about here. In fact, attempting to change your genetic predisposition may actually sabotage our goal of keeping you young.

1.4.4   The PingLongevity™ Test

These are sets of diagnostic tests that we recommend people undergo in PingLongevity™. As medical technology evolves, there will be new tests available and then our list will be continuously revised.

1.4.4.1 Eight Fundamental TCM Tests

On the next page, you'll see a set of simple TCM (Traditional Chinese Medicine) tests to diagnose your internal imbalance through a set of observed symptoms and signs. They correspond to major organ meridian systems and can indicate if you are at risk for disease. In Chapter 5, we'll tell you how you can use some basic TCM formulas to get yourself back in balance based on your test results.

1.4.4.2 Annual Medical Tests

Shown on page 23, these are important tests to help you track your biomarkers several ways. As mentioned in Sections 1.4.1 and 1.4.2, the earlier you start tracking your own genetically disposed medical

EIGHT FUNDAMENTAL TRADITIONAL CHINESE MEDICINE TESTS

LIVER YIN

Pale complexion
Dark circles under the eyes
Anemia
Scanty menstrual period
Blurred vision
Dry eyes
Ophthalmologic problems
Hair loss
Feeling sleepy all the time
Fatigue and dizziness
Spasm in tendons, muscles
Numb, weak limbs
Pale, dry, brittle nails
Depression, easily emotional

HEART

Short of breath, less energy
Pale or purple tongue
Pale face
Mental tiredness, sighing
Irregular heart beat, palpitation
Shallow voice, no energy
Having appetite with no taste
Spontaneous perspiration
Restless mind, insufficient sleep
Forgetfulness, memory loss

KIDNEY YIN

Cold hands or feet
Incontinence or frequent urination
Weak libido, impotence
Premature ejaculation, infertility
Edema and swelling of legs
Easy to catch cold/asthma
Low back pain and ache
Early menopause

Fear, tension and stress
Dream-disturbed sleep
Shortness of breath and tiredness
Urinary tract, prostate problems
Low immune system

LUNGS

Dry cough
Hoarse and low voice
Dry mouth
Pimples, acne
Facial freckles
Skin disorder and rashes
Constipation and dry stool
Chronic sore throat
Nose, throat, trachea discomfort
Rhinitis, hay fever
Allergy, asthma, dermatitis, hives
Psoriasis

LIVER YANG

Redness, swelling in eyes
Burning sensation of eyes
Bags under the eyes
Trigeminal neuralgia
Migraine headache
Menstrual period headache
Blood pressure above normal
Irritable, angers easily
Weak liver function
Varicose veins
Bloating or full feeling in chest
Tenderness below the ribs
Cholesterol above normal
Difficulty concentrating
Child attention deficiency

DIGESTION

Poor digestion & absorption
Reduced appetite
Morning loose stools, diarrhea
Abdominal distension
Leaky gut
Physical/mental tiredness
Pale lips and tongue
Heavy menstrual bleeding
Muscle pain and weakness
Tooth marks on the edge of tongue

KIDNEY YANG

Night or afternoon sweating
Heat/burning in hands, feet
Canker sore, tongue soreness
Red flush/facial rash
Burning and scanty urine
Hair loss, premature graying
Internal heat, desire cold fluids
Anxiety, nervousness
Decreased memory
Loose teeth
Low back, waist soreness and weakness
Joint and bone weakness
Ear ringing or hearing loss
Insomnia

DETOX

Swollen gums
Dry, cracked lips
Thick coating, dark red tongue
Bad breath
Thirst extreme dry mouth
Craving for cold drinks
Constipation
Heartburn, stomachache

ANNUAL MEDICAL TESTS

INSULIN SENSITIVITY

Glucose Tolerance (OGTT)
  Glucose (Fasting)
  Glucose (1 hour)
  Glucose (2 hour)
  Glucose (3 hour)
  Insulin (1 hour)
  Insulin (2 hour)
  Insulin (3 hour)

CANCER MARKER

PSA (male only)
CA-125 (female only)
CCSA-2
CA-19-9

HORMONE PROFILE

DHEA
IGF-1
Cortisol
Total Testosterone
Free Testosterone
DHT (male only)
Estradiol
Estrone (female only)
Estroiol (female only)
Progesterone
2-hydroxyestrone (female)
16-hydroxyestrone (female)
SHBG
LH (Optional)
FSH (Optional)
TSH
T3, T4 free
T3 (reverse)
25-hydroxy Vitamin D

LIPID/BLOOD CHEMISTRY PROFILE

Total Cholesterol
HDL Cholesterol
LDL Cholesterol
Triglycerides
Cholesterol/HDL Ratio
Estimated CHD Risk
Glucose
Homocysteine

AST
AST (SGOT)
ALT (SGPT)
LDH
Total Bilirubin
Alkaline Phosphatase
Iron

Blood Count
Red Blood Cell Count
White Blood Cell Count
Platelet Count
Hemoglobin
Hematocrit
MCV
MCH
MCHC
Polynucleated Cells
Lymphocytes
Monocytes
Eosinophils
Basophils
Polys (absolute)
Lymphs (absolute)
Monocytes (absolute)
Eos (absolute)
Baso (absolute)
RDW

Kidney Function
BUN
Creatinine
BUN/Creatinine Ratio
Uric Acid

Blood Protein
Total Protein
Albumin
Globulin
Albumin/Globulin Ratio

Blood Mineral Panel
Calcium
Potassium
Phosphorus
Sodium
Chloride
Iron

CARDIOVASCULAR & INFLAMMATION

CRP (High-sensitivity)
PLAC
Fibrinogen
ANA (Antinuclear Antibody)

Lipoprotein
EKG
Echocardiogram

OTHER TESTS

Amino Acid Analysis (serum)
Dark Field Blood Analysis
IgG (154), IgE (30) Food Allergy
MVA (mineral, vitamin, amino acid) urine test
Full Body Ultrasound (including carotid)
Brain Electrical Activity Map (qEEG)

Heavy Metal (Urine)
Parasites
H-Scan
Dexa Scan
X-Ray

BIOMARKER SELF TESTS

	PROCEDURE	RESULTS
Forced Vital Capacity (FVC) Test	Use a spirometer. This is the best predictor of bio-age for humans. The FVC reflects a complex function of the integrity of the whole respiratory system, the chest muscles and diaphragm, the central nervous system control mechanisms, the elasticity of the lungs.	VC declines about 40% linearly between 20 and 70 years of age.
Falling Ruler Test	Have someone dangle a ruler, holding it at the 3-centimeter (12-inch) to 50 cm (18-inch) mark (depending on the size of your ruler). Position your thumb and middl e finger about 8 cm (3 inches) apart at equal distance on either side of the bottom of the ruler (the 0-cm/0-inch mark). As the other person drops the ruler, without warning, catch it between your thumb and finger as quickly as possible, and note where you caught it. Repeat three times and average your scores.	This tests the reaction time. Averages generally go from the 15-cm (6-inch) mark at age 20 to 30, to 25 cm (10 inches) at age 40 to 50. and 30 cm (12 inches) or more at age 60.
Static Balance	Stand on a hard surface (not on a rug), bare feet, close your eyes, and lift your foot about 6 inches off the ground, bending your knee at about a 45-degree angle. How many seconds can you stand this way before falling over? Score = average of three trials.	Bio-age: 4 seconds: 70, 5 seconds: 65, 7 seconds: 60, 8 seconds: 55, 9 seconds: 50, 12 seconds: 45, 16 seconds: 40, 22 seconds 30–35, 28 seconds: 25–30.
Visual Accommodation	To test your visual accommodation, hold this page at arms length and slowly move it toward your eyes until the print suddenly begins to blur (if you wear glasses for distance, you may use them, but do not use reading glasses).	For the average 21-year-old, the blurring point will be about 10 cm (4 inches) from the eyes; at age 30, 13 cm (5 inches); at 40, 23 cm (9 inches); and at 50, 38 cm (15 inches) By the time you're 60, your arms probably aren't long enough to bring it into focus at all.
Skin Elasticity	One of the most visible markers of aging is the skin. Loss of connective tissue in the skin contributes to the sagging and wrinkling that are characteristic of aging. A reliable test of skin elasticity is to pinch the skin on the back of your hand between your thumb and forefinger for five seconds, then see how long it takes to return to normal.	This will take less than a second for most people under 30, and 2 to 5 seconds for those ages 40 to 50. However, by age 60, traces of the skin fold will remain for an average of 10 to 15 seconds, and by age 70, 35 to 55 seconds.

parameters, the better you can understand your own individualized optimal targets. You will see variations and trends develop much earlier than you would if you depended on conventional medicine's normal laboratory ranges. In this case, you can detect a changing trend and correct it immediately so you will always be at your optimal level.

1.4.4.3 Self Test:

These are biomarker tests, as discussed in Section 1.2.1 that you could do for yourself.

Besides the biomarker test shown on page 24, you should also monitor your weight, blood pressure, resting temperature and body composition frequently:

TEST	PROTOCOLS
Weight **% Bodywater** **Visceral Fat** **Muscle Mass** **Bone Mass**	First thing in the morning. Use a high-quality scale which has all the functions. Monitor these parameters frequently.
Metabolic Rate **Resting Pulse Rate** **Resting Temperature**	Before getting out of bed when you first wake up. Use a thermometer under arm. Monitor these parameters frequently.
Acidity **Fasting Saliva pH**	First thing in the morning, prior to brushing teeth, eating or drinking.

1.4.4.4 Hormone Profile Test

As discussed in Section 1.4.1, if you have not baselined your own optimal hormone targets when you were young and healthy, it's very difficult to know your optimal hormone range from your laboratory tests, based on the medical normal range. Therefore, the purpose of the hormone profile test is to provide a qualitative test to identify any symptoms of hormone deficiency or imbalance.

In later chapters, you'll know the importance, as well as the interpretation of these measurements.

FEMALE HORMONE PROFILE

TESTOSTERONE DEFICIENCY

Less motivated in general

Low libido

Less in control

Less energetic

More irritable

Loss of muscle & muscle mass

Memory lapses— forgetfulness

Depression and anxiety

Fatigue—feeling "burned out"

Pubic hair thinning

Gaining fat

Aches and pains— arthritic

TESTOSTERONE EXCESS

Excess facial hair and body hair

Voice becomes deeper and less feminine

Increased acne

More hostile, angry, agitated or aggressive

Oily skin

Loss of scalp hair

Trouble tolerating sugars and carbohydrates

ESTROGEN DOMINANCE

More aches and pains

Dysfunctional uterine bleeding

More inflammation and swelling

More allergies and asthma

More twitches and spasms

Mental fogginess or trouble thinking clearly

More mood swings

More fatigued and tired in the morning

More anxiety

Tender breasts and enlargement

Fibrocystic or lumpy breasts

Mood swings—PMS

Water retention

Weight gain—hip area

Cold hands and feet

Cyclical headaches- migraines

Cystic ovaries— polycystic ovaries

Heavy menses

Sleep disturbances— insomnia

Sugar cravings— hypoglycemia

Elevated triglycerides

Infertility or early pregnancy miscarriage

ESTROGEN DEFICIENCY

Hot flashes and night sweats

Low libido, less sensual

Lack of energy

Sleep disturbances

Forgetful

Vaginal dryness & irritation

Bone loss

Incontinence or urinary stress

More wrinkles around mouth and eyes, poor skin tone

Breasts shrinking and sagging

Foggy thinking—unable to focus

Tearfulness

Frequent bladder infections

Heart palpitations

Joint pain, swelling, stiffness

Intolerant to exercise

Painful intercourse

Rapid pulse rate

Dry eyes and dry skin

Loss of sense of well- being

Osteoarthritis

Low total cholesterol

MALE HORMONE PROFILE TEST

(DUE TO DECREASED TESTOSTERONE, AND INCREASED ESTROGEN, DHT, AND SHBG)

Low sex drive	Forgetfulness
Smaller erection angle	Foggy thinking
Less morning un-stimulated erection	Less concentration
Decreased muscle size/tone/strength	Depression and anxiety
Increased abdominal fat	Easily irritated and angry
Prostate enlargement	Decrease in competitiveness
Growth of breasts	Arthritis
Loss of scalp hair	Incontinence
Increased hair in nose, ears, other places	Diabetic
Thinning and drier skin	Bone loss
Lack of energy	Heart disease
Decreased flexibility	Low DHEA
Aches and pains	Sleep disturbances

1.5   SUMMARY

The following gives you an outline of what we have covered in this chapter:

- PingLongevity™ is a way of life to keep you 20 to 30 years younger than your chronological age both internally and externally. Our goal is to slow down your rate of aging by half, and extend your productive years by as much as 50%.

- There is no one-pill-fixes-all solution to slow, stop and reverse aging, as well as extend life. You must practice a complete and holistic solution, covered by PingLongevity™ protocols in the following chapters.

- Your ideal or normal range of medical tests is the same as those when you were 18 to 22 years old or as close to it as possible to a time in when you were young and healthy. This will be used to compare your trends and allow intervention to reset your body back your ideal. Therefore, it is vital to perform a set of comprehensive tests annually to track your body's status.

CHAPTER 2

The Science of Food

D o you eat a typical American breakfast? You know what I mean —bacon and/or sausage, eggs, fried potatoes, toast, butter, jam, juice.

What if you could eat a breakfast that is a nutrition powerhouse by comparison: Approximately 40% lower in calories, 86% less saturated fat, 650% more omega-3 fatty acids, 99% less cholesterol, 5000 oxygen radical absorbance capacity (ORAC), loads of vitamins and minerals from super green vegetables and loads of natural food enzymes.

What if you eat this new breakfast day in and day out? Don't you think you'll be miles ahead in the journey toward a healthier, more vibrant, and longer life?

We are not dreaming here. The special breakfast we are talking about is referred to as the PingLongevity™ Mix. It is a very condensed nutritionally rich mix that our clinic patients have been using for years. See the following page for a detailed comparison with a typical breakfast.

There are so many kinds of diets: Atkins, South Beach, Mediterranean, Zone, Low Carb, UltraSimple, Full Plate, Kind Diet, Eat-Clean, Flat-Belly, Mayo Clinic, Perfect 10, Fat Resistance, American Heart Association, American Diabetic Association, just to name a few. Which one should you follow?

There are also many gurus, experts, nutritionists and doctors offering food advice, but are they offering you valid information?

TYPICAL BREAKFAST

	CALORIES	SATURATED FAT (G)	OMEGA 3	OTHER FAT (G)	PROTEIN (G)	CHOLESTEROL (MG)
2 scrambled eggs	202.0	4.5	—	10.4	13.5	430.0
1 cup of whole milk	146.0	5.0	0.1	2.9	8.0	24.0
1 cup of canned orange juice	112.0	0.1	—	0.5	1.7	0.0
1 breakfast Tarantino sausage	90.0	3.0	—	7.0	7.0	30.0
2 slice of white bread	132.0	0.4	—	1.3	3.8	0.0
Total (*Source:* FatSecret)	682.0	12.9	0.1	22.1	34.1	484.0
PINGLONGEVITY™ MIX						
3 tsp raw milled chia seeds	50.0	0.4	3.0	1.0	3.0	0.0
3 tsp raw milled wheatgerm	36.0	0.0	0.4	0.4	2.3	0.0
3 tsp raw milled flaxseeds	30.0	0.2	2.0	0.5	1.3	0.0
2 tsp raw wolfberry & He Shou Wu mix	25.0	0.0	0.0	0.0	0.8	0.0
1 cup raw organic fat free milk (or raw almond milk)	86.0	0.3	0.0	0.6	8.4	5.0
5 walnuts	130.0	1.2	1.0	10.8	3.1	0.0
1 tsp vegetable powder	12.0	0.0	—	1.0	1.0	0.0
1 tsp high ORAC fruit powder	20.0	0.0	—	1.0	1.0	0.0
2 tsp of protein powder	40.0	0.0	—	0.2	6.7	0.0
Total	429.0	2.1	6.4	15.5	27.5	5.0
PingLongevity™ Mix as % of Typical Breakfast	63%	16%	6440%	70%	81%	1%

- When Yahoo Healthy Living tells you that McDonald's small French fries are healthier than others, should you go pick up the fries?

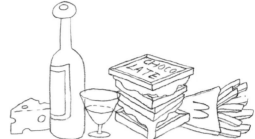

- When it tells you that chocolate is healthy, are you free to eat it without knowing the sugar and flavonol contents?

- When people tell you to drink red wine every night, because of resveratrol and flavonoids, should you go ahead and drink it without knowing the negative effects of alcohol?

The multitude of diets and conflicting advice is certainly confusing. In fact, when you probe a little deeper, much diet advice is either biased or incomplete. For example:

- Few diet plans talk about how foods should be prepared. A healthy whole-grain food can easily be reduced to simple sugar by high temperature cooking. A good protein and fatty-acid food can easily become carcinogenic if it is cooked at a high temperature.

- Many of the diet plans oppose the use of carbohydrates. However, the high protein and fats intake they promote are much less efficient sources of fuel for the body.

- A very high protein and fat diet puts a lot of unnecessary stress on the liver and kidneys.

- Many carbohydrates may have a low glycemic index if prepared correctly.

- A complete healthy diet must consist of foods that are alkaline forming, enzyme rich, nutritionally dense and low glycemic. In addition, no diet can be healthy without having the correct water, juice, drink, supplementation and food order. No diet can be healthy without a good food combination of proteins, carbohydrates and fat prepared in a specific manner.

In this chapter, we'll discuss extensively the science of food, put in practice in the PingLongevity™ Diet.

2.1   RAW FOOD AND ENZYME POTENTIAL

"Each one of us is given a limited supply of bodily enzyme energy at birth. This supply, like the energy supply in your new battery, has to last a lifetime. The faster you use up your enzyme supply, the shorter your life. A great deal of our enzyme energy is wasted haphazardly throughout life. The habit of cooking our food and eating it processed with chemicals and the use of alcohol, drugs and junk food all draw out tremendous quantities of enzymes from our limited supply. Frequent colds and fevers and exposure to extremes of temperature also deplete the supply. A body in such a weakened, enzyme-deficient state is a prime target for cancer, obesity, heart disease or other degenerative problems. A lifetime of such abuse often ends in the tragedy of death at middle age."

—Dr. Edward Howell

Many "experts" offer advice on eating healthy foods such as whole grains, vegetables and fruits. They also single out special high-nutrient foods like oats.

However, they often are ignorant about food preparation. Any great whole food can be reduced to an unhealthy food by cooking. A not-so-high temperature above 118 degrees Fahrenheit can effectively kill all the natural enzymes in foods. A higher temperature can destroy many nutrients. An even higher temperature can break down complex carbohydrates into simple sugars (or starch). So you'd think oats, or beans, or sweet potatoes or whole grains are good stuff. But when you cook them into starchy form, they lose most of their nutritional value. Similarly, raw vegetables are very nutritious. But through cooking, they become starchy and lose many of their nutrients and all their enzymes.

2.1.1 Human Enzyme Potential

Living things constantly undergo chemical processes including burning energy, storing energy, synthesizing protein, breaking down food, expelling toxins, making new cells and repairing damaged DNA. We all have the machinery needed to liberate and store chemical energy from foods and to create complex molecules from simpler ones for the building of new structures. These processes collectively are called metabolism and involve the transformation by enzyme-catalyzed reactions of both matter and energy.

Enzymes, a form of protein, are the chemical agents necessary for every chemical reaction to take place in your body. Without enzymes, all bodily functions come to a stop: There is no energy production, no muscle contraction, no breathing, no digestion.

According to the ancient law of living, every living thing has a fixed energy potential. Similarly, modern scientists believe our total enzyme potential is limited. During our lifetimes, we are capable of producing only a certain amount of enzymes. When there are insufficient enzymes in the body, many critical chemical reactions, such as cell repair, don't occur efficiently or don't occur at all. As a result, the body becomes diseased and aging is accelerated. The faster we produce and use up enzymes, the faster we age.

Thus, metabolism is the sum of all life processes and enzymes are the agents of all metabolism. Without enzymes, we simply die. A key to vibrant health and long life is to preserve the body's limited number of enzymes as long as possible. One way to do this is to eat natural food that has its own enzymes so we don't have to expend our own supply of enzymes to digest our food.

2.1.2 Enzymes in Raw Foods

Digestive enzymes help break down food into usable nutrients and fuels. They are found in saliva, pancreatic secretions and digestive fluids found in the stomach and small intestine. Today it is easy to waste a large amount of our total enzyme potential on producing digestive enzymes because the food we consume has so little enzyme content of its own. By depending on the enzymes already in our food, it is possible to save up to 50% of our body's digestive enzymes.

We eat living things (plants and animals) and take in air (oxygen) to absorb the necessary fuel (calories) and nutrients for sustaining life. By nature's design, every living thing has its own specialized chemicals, called food enzymes, to decompose itself at the proper temperature and moisture levels. Food enzymes are destroyed at a temperature above 118°F and are usually most effective at around 98°F with the correct moisture conditions. True, 118°F is below the generally recommended temperature for cooking food. On the other hand, a moist 98°F equals conditions in the human stomach, where food is pre-digested.

Therefore, *every living thing contains the exact food enzyme to decompose itself under optimal conditions—and these conditions are identical to the natural environment of the human digestive tract. We are in tune with this law of food when we eat food in a state where its enzymes are alive.*

Some foods are supposed to be eaten raw and fresh because that is when they are enzyme rich. Another way to keep a food's natural enzyme alive is to prepare it pickled, sprouted, low-temperature smoked or naturally dried.

In the old teachings of Traditional Chinese Medicine, it is not considered a good idea to eat "raw cold" food. Many people, even TCM doctors, wrongly understand to mean we shouldn't eat raw food. Actually, the Chinese word "raw cold" can also mean "immature" or "unripe." For example, the enzymes in unripe raw fruits are in an inactive state. When fruit is ripe, due to enzyme activities, the fruits become soft. If left alone, in warm damp climate, it will be spoiled because it is being digested by its own enzymes. Therefore, TCM promotes eating ripe foods when they are rich in food enzymes.

In some foods, we need to be careful about enzyme inhibitors.

Some raw foods, like seeds and nuts, have their enzymes naturally locked due to the need for storage in order to be able to sprout at the appropriate time in nature. Therefore, a much longer time is needed, under the right temperature and moisture conditions, for their enzymes to become active. This is because they contain a substance called an enzyme inhibitor, which keeps the enzymes from being effective in the food's raw state.

Because their food enzymes are inactive, raw grains and seeds are difficult for us to digest. Our bodies need to produce additional digestive enzymes to enable us to break down the enzymes in raw foods. After wild food became less available, early man learned to farm and cook grains. But the cooking process destroys the food's enzymes.

The best way for us to unlock the enzyme inhibitors in grains and seeds and still preserve their natural enzymes is to eat grains and seeds in a sprouted or fermented state. This is how chickens, birds, and squirrels eat them. A chicken, for example, has a craw, a sort of pre-stomach, which stores grains for days and causes it to ferment before real digestion. Squirrels bury seeds until they sprout. Then they dig out the seed and eat the tender sprout. In both cases, living food is eaten in its natural state and digestion depends on natural enzymes—the food's own chemicals of decomposition.

Another way to take advantage of the enzyme power in grains and seeds is to eat them when they are very young. Very young corn, for example, can be eaten raw because it is so soft and milky inside.

2.1.3 Live Energy in Raw Foods

According to the universal law of energy (more about this in Chapter 10), the higher the frequency at which energy vibrates, the closer it is to the ultimate Tao, the infinite energy source. Applied to humans, the higher one's Chi and spirit energy, the more we can "communicate" to the cosmic energy sources to extend our own energy level and life. *Thus, the highest energy source is the subtle energy from the universe. The more we can access and absorb this energy, the more we can preserve our own energy.* Higher beings (people with more pure energy) are able to absorb this higher subtle energy from the universe.

Modern science and medicine have only emphasized the need for "nutrition" from the physical constituents of the food because they cannot measure or understand higher energy. While the physical nutrients are important, they are a lower form of energy compared to the food's higher energy of chi and spirit.

All living things possess the higher energy of chi and spirit, which is attached to the living form. When the physical form dies, the higher energy disperses. When we consume food in its natural state, we can absorb its higher energy. For example, when a living thing, such as an apple, dies, the higher energy leaves its physical form. When we consume food in its natural state, fresh and raw, we also absorb its higher energy, which cannot be measured by modern instruments.

Food produces energy at different levels. We are not just talking about the calories and nutrients for the measurable energy needs of the body, but also higher subtle energy forms. To repeat, cooked food has less of this higher energy than raw, fresh, or live food. These live foods receive energy from the universe (for example, in the form of sunlight, which is yang energy) and from the earth (such as in the form of nutrients, which is yin energy) and synthesize them into energy that humans can absorb.

In summary, food has three values to humans: (1) calories to burn to produce energy for work, such as thinking and walking; (2) nutrition to nourish the body for such things as building and repairing tissues; and (3) higher level energy, the chi, to sustain life.

All natural foods in their raw living states have these three values. Modern processed foods, however, are high in calories, but low in nutrition and energy. When we eat a lot of processed food, we tend to eat more because the value of the food cannot satisfy our bodies' needs.

2.1.4   Raw Foods: A Way of Eating

If you grew up in the countryside, you may have the opportunity to dig out sweet potatoes and eat them raw right there in the fields. You may notice that they are not as sweet and not starchy at all when eaten raw as compared with baked ones. In addition, it takes much longer to eat because you really have to chew it well before taking it in. Therefore, when we follow what God gives to us in its natural way, we'll have to eat slowly so that the food goes through the digestive processes of saliva and chewing.

Can you chew gum and recover more quickly from colon surgery? This is exactly what was found by a study performed by a team of British researchers. "Chewing gum may speed the return of normal bowel function after colon surgery. Some patients have trouble moving their bowels after colon surgery, but chewing gum may fool the body into good digestion."

It's an interesting discovery. It supports major elements of healthy eating. The PingLongevity™ Diet cares about not only what you eat, but also how you prepare and eat the food. This is because a good healthy food can become unhealthy if you do not cook it right and eat it correctly.

Nature has made most raw foods such that you have to really chew them thoroughly before you can swallow them, moving them into the stomach and digestive tract.

For example, let's eat raw vegetables and well-cooked vegetables side-by-side. The cooked ones can be chewed and swallowed at least twice as fast as the raw ones. Another example: Let's compare eating cooked versus raw sweet potatoes. You simply cannot send the raw ones into your stomach unless you chew at least five times the amount of time as the cooked ones. This would force you to pre-digest the food very well. According to the above discovery, it not only helps digestion, but also helps bowel function.

We actually eat smaller quantities of raw foods than cooked foods because when the food is less starchy, it is harder to eat, giving us a chance to feel satisfied without eating too much.

When we eat raw foods, we also feel like we have eaten a large quantity of food. This is easily verified. Just do an experiment: Take one bowl of vegetables and cook it. See how much the volume shrinks. So when you eat raw, you have taken in a larger volume for the same calories.

Many raw protein foods are much easier to digest than cooked ones. For example, raw fish, shrimp, meat are much softer than cooked ones. Protein and fat become harder when processed at a high temperature. I often hear people marvel at the dish on the dinner table in a fine restaurant, "Wow, the fish is so soft," usually demonstrating the skill of the chef. I wonder if they ever think about how soft the raw sashimi tuna is.

2.1.5 Processed Foods, Enzymes and Degenerative Diseases

The so-called advancement of civilization has addressed the issue of hunger through new technologies of food processing so that harvested foods can be stored for a long time and transported for long distances. Unfortunately, most of the processing removes the effect of food enzymes.

For example, in order to mass produce, store and market food products, all enzymes and bacteria must be killed. In response to the need to store food for long periods of time, the food industry cooks, pasteurizes (milk, fruit juice) and processes (packaged vegetables). This usually involves high temperature cooking and the addition of preservatives.

As a consequence of eating foods prepared in this way, more and more people are overweight and are plagued by degenerative diseases. We have developed a body system that adapts to enzyme-less food, so our systems are forced to produce huge amounts of digestive enzymes. Because so much of our enzyme potential is used to produce digestive enzymes, our capability for producing enzymes for other metabolic functions, such as maintaining a strong immune system and cell rebuilding, has become deficient. This is one of the reasons wildlife in their natural habitat do not suffer from degenerative diseases. They usually die only when killed by predators, natural disasters and contagious diseases caused by deadly epidemics.

Modern man has greatly accelerated the rate of enzyme depletion. It becomes obvious that eating food in its raw state or in a state that keeps food enzymes alive (pickled, sprouted, low-temperature smoked, naturally dried) will dramatically preserve the body's enzyme essence, reduce the rate of aging and prevent or delay degenerative diseases.

Another major reason for food processing, we are told, is to avoid deadly bacteria in foods. It is as though eating processed food is safer because it is totally sterilized. We city people are afraid of drinking natural water and eating raw foods in a remote village. But why are the locals healthy and with fewer degenerative diseases?

We visited the remote East African Masai tribe. We wanted to study every culture. How do they eat, drink and exercise? How long they live? Do they have degenerative diseases?

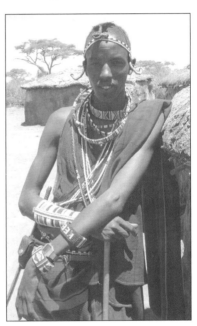

Typical Masai tribesman

These are among the healthiest people in the world. They drink fresh raw milk and fresh raw live blood from their cows. Once in a while, they eat meat. They never eat any vegetables or fruits. Of course, their cows get all the fruit and vegetable nutrients in their milk and blood! Many of the degenerative diseases are unheard of among the Masai. They are super healthy, athletic and slim.

We also met some Masai who worked in the nearby five-star resort where we stayed. Many Masai, after working in the hotel and eating the more Westernized food for one year, become overweight and some are starting to show signs of diabetes.

What a dramatic demonstration of the concept you are indeed what you eat!

Up until 2009, we were able to buy raw milk in health food stores in California, under a "pet food" license. The FDA decided to make the sale of raw milk unlawful because we humans created too much demand.

Nowadays you are told to avoid bacteria at all costs, namely by eating sterile foods (pasteurized). Here is what a typical government health bulletin tells you:

> "Pasteurized juice is safe because it has been heated hot enough and long enough to kill bacteria.
>   Pasteurization is the process of heating liquid or semi-liquid foods to a particular temperature for a designated period sufficient to destroy certain bacteria."
>   —BOULDER COUNTY COLORADO GOVERNMENT ONLINE

Don't you know that bacteria are around us everywhere, on our hands, mouths, inside our bodies? If we can eat raw fruits, why do we have to drink pasteurized fruit juice because of the scary bacteria?

The key is not to get you sterile, but rather to have a healthy immune system! When we are too much into sterile (pasteurized) food, we kill the digestive enzymes (life force) in the food. Studies show the lack of digestive enzymes in our food is a major cause of aging and degenerative diseases.

By the way, if you see a bottle of fruit juice in the supermarket labeled "100% fruit juice," it's almost sure that the juice is pasteurized and made from concentrates. The result is longer shelf life, not a longer and younger life for you!

Modern food producing industries hand-in-hand with government regulatory agencies, teach people to be afraid of the same bacteria that occur naturally all around us. They make sure all foods we eat are highly processed through pasteurization, not only for dairy products, but also for fruit and vegetable juices.

Indeed through processing, they kill all germs and prevent a tiny percent chance of people accidentally dying of bacterial infection. By doing this, they have created foods that are depleted in live food digestive enzymes and other essential nutrients—the very life force that is essential to health!

The tradeoff is either to have millions of people who have degenerative diseases due to lowered body enzyme potential resulting in an inability to absorb nutrients and a reduced immune system that is incapable of dealing with normal environmental bacteria or to risk a tiny number of bacterial infections, insignificant compared to the rate of degenerative diseases. This makes us wonder, is the rationale really for food preservation and profitability of the processed food industry or for the true benefit of consumers?

2.1.6   Now Let's Test Our IQ

Are the following foods healthy, as the experts have told you?

- Tuna fish is healthy. Therefore, whenever we go to Subway, we pick up a tuna fish sandwich. Is it healthy? Not necessarily! You are eating very high temperature processed canned food. You're also getting highly processed mayonnaise and bread. You may also be exposed to heavy metals.

- Fruit is good. Let's take a look at pasteurized fruit juice and canned fruits, like what's usually on the breakfast table. Is this healthy? Definitely not! These processed foods are poor in nutrition, deprived of food enzymes and full of sugar.

- Milk and dairy products are nutritious. Let's take pasteurized milk. Healthy? Not! They are actually sources of allergy and indigestion.

- Vegetables are healthy, but not if you eat fully cooked ones because you have eliminated all enzymes and lots of nutrients.

- Is whole grain good? Some grains are very nutritious, but most of the time, the standard cooking/processing converts them to starchy simple sugars.

- Protein and certain fatty acids are essential for a healthy diet. But what about exposing them to high temperatures in cooking? It will turn good oils to bad ones.

- Is boiling food good? After all it avoids using oils, right? According to University of Wisconsin, *Journal of Home Economics*, Vol. 17, N.5, boiling foods can result in a major mineral loss:

Mineral	Boiling	Pressure Cooking
Iron	49.0%	17.4%
Calcium	31.0%	12.0%
Phosphorus	46.4%	19.4%
Magnesium	44.7%	21.1%

Nuts are very nutritious food. Right? Wait, let's hear the story of Dan:

"During the last annual physical, I was shocked to find that my trans fat levels were high, although I never eat anything close to trans fat.

Upon investigation, I finally zoomed in on a few boxes of very delicious oil-free, salt-free peanuts that a friend of mine sent to me. Once I got started with these peanuts, I could not stop. They were so delicious and crispy. It would not take much time for me to consume a whole box. I knew I should not eat too many nuts at one time because of calories. However, my excuse was at least it's healthily cooked.

Well, as I dug deeper, I wondered why I was not so addicted to the home roasted peanuts. They don't really taste that great. The nutmeat is more oily (non-crispy) and bitter. I suddenly realized that to make the delicious nuts crispy, the manufacturer must put the nuts through a high temperature drying process. Oils, especially polyunsaturated oils, may oxidize and hydrogenate under really high temperatures. Indeed, nature makes foods that naturally limit your appetite. Humans have learned to process delicious unhealthy foods that can greatly increase your appetite."

—DAN, BEVERLY HILLS

We can give endless examples. It's critical to remember the principle of raw food: enzymes and live energy. Dr. Walter Last, a raw food guru summarized it well:

The main biochemical and nutritional benefit of eating raw foods as compared to cooked foods:

- A higher vitamin and mineral content;

- Minerals are largely present as biologically active colloids;

- An abundance of helpful enzymes and bio-energy or life-force;

- Proteins remain in their natural condition instead of being denatured;

- The absence of digestive leukocytosis, an increase of white blood cells in affected organs in response to infection or toxins. This also occurs when we eat cooked food. The intestinal wall becomes flooded with white blood cells but this does not happen when eating raw food. The higher the food has been heated, the stronger is the leukocytosis and the more toxic is this food for our body;

- Polyunsaturated fatty acids and cholesterol do not become oxidized and carcinogenic or atherogenic;

- Glucose is absorbed more slowly, protecting blood-sugar regulation;

- There is no overweight or obesity on a raw food diet;

- As counted in calories, much less food is required;

- Proven cleansing, rejuvenating and anti-cancer properties

2.2   LOW GLYCEMIC INDEX FOODS

Living whole foods, including fruits, fish, beans, seeds and unprocessed meat of different textures and flavors are digested slowly in the human body because some parts of them are not quickly decomposable. Take wheat for example: Whole wheat contains germ, endosperm and bran. We humans think it's too difficult to digest, so we refine it. Refined wheat has only endosperm, the most refined sugar like starchy part, which digests very fast. Nature's wild animals have their systems tuned to digesting food slowly over many hours. Thus, living whole food is meant to be digested slowly, little by little. When we eat foods that are slower to digest, we get more benefit from the food.

2.2.1   Insulin Sensitivity

Civilization has made giant steps in refining foods, such as making flours refined from grains, pure oil from beans, salt from natural sea salt and sugar from canes. Advanced methods also synthesize several refined foods into one product. When we eat refined food, we digest it within a couple of hours or even faster, using lots of enzymes produced by our bodies rather than the food's natural enzymes (which act more slowly).

Starch is a good example: The starch in raw food is stored in hard, compact granules, which are difficult to digest quickly. During cooking at high temperatures, water and heat cause the starch granules to expand, burst and free up individual molecules. This is how gravy is made—by heating flour and water until the starch granules burst and the gravy thickens. Cooking starchy food makes it much easier and faster to digest, but this creates other challenges for the body.

Quickly digested food is broken down into simple sugar, which in turn floods into the bloodstream. When blood sugar peaks, the pancreas releases insulin to store energy and to convert unused energy to fat. Insulin also inhibits the burning of already existing fat. When there is a sharp increase in blood sugar, a large quantity of insulin is released by the pancreas. The insulin does its work and makes the blood sugar drop. But this sudden drop in blood sugar then makes us hungry, so we crave more food. Thus, accelerated digestion causes three unhealthy patterns:

- High insulin assists conversion of sugar into fat and inhibits the burning of fat. That's a reason that sometimes even if you starve yourself, you still don't lose weight.

- The quick drop in blood sugar, due to a violent insulin response, generates a craving for more food and thus more calorie intake. The cycle continues.

- Fast digestion makes the body adapt to eating food that has no enzymes of its own. The body makes up the difference and becomes a digestive enzyme-making machine. This not only reduces the amount of enzymes that are available for other metabolic functions but it also speeds up the depletion of our total enzyme potential.

On the other hand, when we eat foods that are digested more slowly, we reverse these unhealthy patterns. *Slower digestion, or more precisely, a slower release of sugar into the bloodstream, makes us less hungry, burns more fat and teaches the body to wait for the food's own enzymes to take action.*

Eating food that digests slowly also keeps our blood sugar and insulin response as smooth and even as possible. The standard glucose tolerance test (GTT) measures the body's response to an oral dose of glucose. The patient must fast for 12 hours prior to the test. A baseline fasting blood sugar and insulin are measured. Then a glucose-rich drink (glucola) is administered. After ingesting the "cola," blood sugar and insulin are measured at 30, 60, 90, and 120 minutes. The following diagram, from "The Role of Dietary Carbohydrate in the Decreased Glucose Tolerance of the Elderly," an article published in the 1987 *Journal of American Geriatrics*, shows the typical glucose-insulin response for healthy young people versus old people.

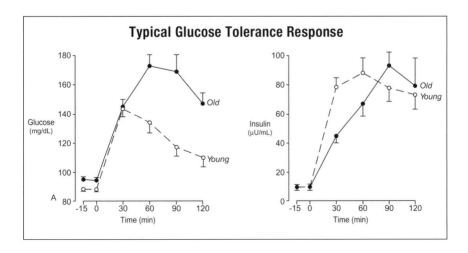

"Eric, a patient at the clinic, has been on the PingLongevity™ Diet for several years. At age 45, by eating a slow digesting, live-enzyme food and by following a caloric-restriction diet, he can achieve a fasting glucose between 60 and 85, and then can return to exactly the same level 120 minutes after taking glu-cola. By comparison, 120 minutes after consuming the glucola drink, a young healthy individual on a normal diet can only return his glucose levels to 115, a level far higher than the start-ing baseline glucose of 90 (measured when fasting)."

—Dr. Ping

2.2.2   The Glycemic Index

The scientific method of measuring the absorption rate of food into the bloodstream is known as the glycemic index (GI), which is the ratio of absorption rates between a particular food and pure sugar, both containing equivalent amounts of carbohydrates. Pure sugar is the easiest to absorb and therefore has a rating of 100. The index of any food is less or equal to 100 (%). The higher the index, the quicker the food is absorbed into the bloodstream. *To increase our longevity and our health, we should eat food with a lower glycemic index, the low GI foods.*

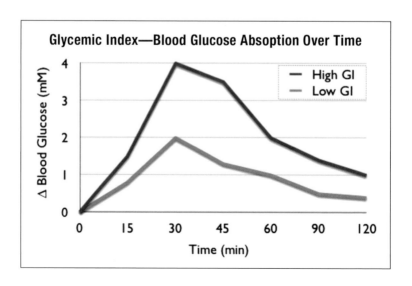

In general, starchy and refined foods have a higher glycemic index because they are easily decomposed into the blood. Proteins, fat and whole foods have a lower index. A low GI food mixed with high one can generally lower the GI. For example, pasta is made of mixing oil with flours. It has relatively lower GI, although flour has high one. Below is a list of very low and very high GI foods:

GLYCEMIC INDEX OF FOODS

VEGETABLES		DAIRY	
Soybeans	18	Non-fat plain yogurt	14
Broccoli, cauliflower, celery	10–25	Whole milk	27
Beans	27–48	Ice cream, vanilla	61
Sweet corn	48		
French fries, baked	54	**FRUITS**	
Beets	64	Grapefruit	25
Potato, peeled & steamed	65	Apple	38
		Orange	44
GRAINS		Grapes, green	46
Peanuts	14	Kiwi	52
Whole-grain bread	40	Banana	55
Linguine	40	Mango	55
Rye bread	50	Watermelon	72
Brown rice, steamed	50		
White bread	70	**DRINK**	
White rice	72	Apple juice	40
		Fruit punch	67
MEATS		Cola	77
Sausages	28	Gatorade	78
Lean chicken	36		
Fish strips	38	**OTHER**	
Beef casserole	53	Vinegar	0

2.2.3   Carbohydrate, Protein, and Fat

Many experts urge you to stay away from carbohydrates, and eat a predominantly protein and fat diet. They figured that carbohydrates have a high glycemic index, while proteins and fat have lower ones. Therefore, carbohydrate is the culprit of making you fat.

This is completely missing the mark.

First, not all carbohydrates have a high glycemic index. Glancing the table in section 2.2.2, you'll see a lot of fruits and vegetables are, in fact, lower on the glycemic index than meats and fats. Many grains, such as quinoa, flaxseed, sesame, wheat germ and chia are low glycemic index. However, if these grains are refined, they may become high glycemic.

Second, our bodies not only need nutrition from foods, but also energy to support the work we do everyday, including basic metabolic functions. Carbohydrates are the body's most efficient fuel. They can easily convert to glucose (blood sugar) and readily be utilized as fuel by the cells. On the other hand, proteins and fat, as energy forms, are not the most efficient.

Third, carbohydrates also provide basic cell functions such as cell-to-cell communications.

What is the function of fat in the body? In nature, animals accumulate fat as energy reserves to keep them from starving, because food is sometimes unavailable for a long period of time. Bears accumulate lots of fat before winter and slowly burn it off during hibernation. Thus, fat is used to store energy during periods of no energy intake.

We need a continuous supply of glucose in the bloodstream to carry out all the body's functions and to supply tissues with energy. If you're dieting or starving, when glucose intake is low, your liver supplies a very limited reserve of energy. After that, many tissues switch over to use the products of fat breakdown (known as ketones) as an alternative source of fuel. When glucose is scarce, ketones are produced from fatty tissue and transported through the bloodstream to the liver, where ketone bodies are formed. The ketone bodies are then released into the bloodstream to be taken up and used for energy by the muscles, heart, brain and many other tissues.

Like cars, our bodies can use different types of fuels. Cars use diesel, regular, unleaded or supreme unleaded gasoline. Regular gasoline burns far less efficiently than supreme grade, leaving more oxidation and waste products inside the car engines. Similarly, burning ketones from fat is a much less efficient process than burning glucose, leaving more oxidants or free radicals in the body. The result: The body ages more quickly.

Therefore, we do need carbohydrates in our diet. We need good carbohydrates, namely complex ones, not simple sugars (e.g., starchy food).

In a developed nation such as the United States, there is almost always more food than we can consume. Fat in our bodies has, in fact, lost its use. We should be thinner and yet 61% of Americans are overweight. Why? Because the food we eat has a high glycemic index and a high insulin sensitivity. When insulin is high, fat is not burned. A person becomes hungrier and wants to eat more. When there is a constant need to produce a high quantity of insulin, the body either begins to lose the ability to produce more insulin or becomes less effective in binding insulin to cell receptors, resulting in diabetes. Type 2 diabetes is poised to strike about 33% of adult Americans by 2050, according to the latest statistics of U.S. Centers of Disease Control and Prevention.

2.3   ALKALINE FORMING FOODS

The measure of the acidity or alkalinity of a media is called pH. It is measured on a scale of 0 to 14. The media is neutral at 7.0, acidic when below 7.0 and alkaline when above 7.0.

Our bodies need to maintain a very tight alkaline blood pH value in order to survive. In healthy people, the pH of blood is around 7.4.

The body is constantly bombarded with acid forming substances, increasingly so in an industrialized world. All metabolic waste products are acidic. Nearly all processed foods are acidic. For example, soft drinks like Coke are acidic. It takes 32 bottles of eight-ounce pH-9 alkaline water to neutralize one can of Coke's acidity. If you soak a baby tooth in a can of soda, it will disappear in 8 hours and a T-bone from a T-bone steak will be dissolved in two and a half days.

In order to maintain blood at near constant pH, the body keeps an alkaline reserve. When needed, alkaline minerals such as calcium are drawn from joints, bones and other tissues into the bloodstream, neutralizing extra acidity.

The pH of saliva parallels the extracellular fluid, the most consistent and most definitive physical sign of the ionic calcium deficiency syndrome. It is scientifically documented that up to 150 diseases are related to calcium deficiency and overacidity of the body system.

2.3.1   Food Alkalinity and Acidity

Foods are digested and broken down into either an acid or an alkaline end product in the body. This end product is called the "ash" and is what remains in the body after the food has been broken down.

Foods that leave alkaline ash after digestion are called "alkaline-forming foods." On the other hand, those producing acid ash are called "acid-forming" foods.

It's important to note that food pH and its "ash" pH may be quite different. For example: lemons, limes and grapefruits taste tart and are chemically acid, but tests show that when they are metabolized in the body they actually have an alkalizing effect, hence alkaline-forming.

On the other hand, meat tests alkaline before digestion, but leaves very acidic residue in the body. Therefore, it is acid forming.

Examples of acid forming foods are meat, sugars, eggs and dairy and most grains, white flour and carbonated beverages. Pharmaceuticals are acid forming. Artificial chemical sweeteners like NutraSweet and Equal (asparatme) are extremely acid forming.

Fresh fruits and vegetables are alkaline forming in the body and contain many electrolyte minerals that help to maintain a healthy pH balance of 7.4 and a reserve of critical electrolytes.

On the following page is a food table of alkaline- and acid-forming foods.

Some of you may not be able to tolerate acid tasting, alkaline-forming foods.

FOOD ALKALINE/ACID FORMING TABLE

CATEGORY	STRONG ALKALINE	ALKALINE	WEAK ALKALINE	ACID	WEAK ACID	STRONG ACID
Sweeteners			Raw Honey, Raw Sugar	Processed Honey, Molasses	White Sugar, Brown Sugar	NutraSweet, Equal, Aspartame, Sweet 'n Low
Fruits	Lemons, Watermelon, Limes, Grapefruit, Mangoes, Papayas	Dates, Figs, Melons, Grapes, Papaya, Kiwi, Berries, Apples, Pears, Raisins	Oranges, Bananas, Cherries, Pineapple, Peaches, Avocadoes	Plums, Processed Fruit Juices	Sour Cherries, Rhubarb	Blueberries, Cranberries, Prunes
Beans Vegetables Legumes	Asparagus, Onions, Vegetable Juices, Raw Parsley, Raw Spinach, Broccoli, Garlic	Okra, Squash, Green Beans, Beets, Celery, Lettuce, Zucchini, Sweet Potato, Carob	Carrots, Tomatoes, Fresh Corn, Mushrooms, Cabbage, Peas, Potato Skins, Olives, Soybeans, Tofu	Cooked Spinach, Kidney Beans, String Beans	Potatoes (without skins), Pinto Beans, Navy Beans, Lima Beans	Chocolate
Nuts Seeds		Almonds	Chestnuts	Pumpkin Seeds, Sunflower Seeds	Pecans, Cashews	Peanuts, Walnuts
Oils		Flax Seed Oil	Canola Oil	Corn Oil		
Grains Cereals			Amaranth, Millet, Wild Rice, Quinoa	Sprouted Wheat Bread, Spelt, Brown Rice	White Rice, Corn, Buckwheat, Oats, Rye	Wheat, White Flour, Pastries, Pasta
Meats				Venison, Cold Water Fish	Turkey, Chicken, Lamb	Beef, Pork, Shellfish
Eggs Dairy		Breast Milk	Soy Cheese, Soy Milk, Goat Milk, Goat Cheese, Whey	Eggs, Butter, Yogurt, Buttermilk, Cottage Cheese	Raw Milk	Cheese, Homogenized Milk, Ice Cream
Beverages	Herb Teas, Lemon Water	Green Tea	Ginger Tea	Tea	Coffee	Beer, Soft Drinks

"For some people, who suffer from leaky gut syndrome, some acid tasting, but alkaline-forming foods, may cause problems. This is because they cannot digest the foods fully and the foods cannot be converted to alkaline ash yet. The undigested acid is absorbed and becomes a problem. These patients should avoid acid tasting alkaline forming foods, such as citrus, vinegar or even tomatoes."
    —DR. PING

2.3.2   The Body's Alkaline Reserve

In order for the body to maintain a near constant level of pH in the blood, we maintain alkaline reserves, or electrolytes, to combat acidity. When excess acids must be neutralized, alkaline reserves are mobilized.

As you may see from the food table in section 2.3.1, due to the predominance of processed food in our diet, we are increasingly eating a diet that is acid-forming food dominant. As a result, our bodies are deprived of an alkaline buffer and the ability to neutralize the acidity. When this happens, the body either has to get calcium and other alkaline minerals from the bones, losing bone density, or deposit the acid waste in the joints and fat. That's the origin of osteoporosis.

"We have seen many patients with painful, inflamed and swollen finger and thumb joints. Many of them, after eating acid foods, immediately feel pain in these joints. After reducing their intake of acid-forming foods and increasing alkalinity, they find their pain and swelling disappear in a matter of a few days."
    —DR. PING

This condition forces the body to borrow the alkaline minerals such as calcium, sodium, potassium and magnesium from organs and bones to buffer (neutralize) the acid and safely remove it from the body. Because of this strain, the body can suffer severe and prolonged damage due to high acidity, a condition that may go undetected for years.

Studies have consistently shown that heavy consumption of soft drinks pulls minerals out of our bones, causing a loss of huge amounts of calcium, magnesium and other trace minerals into urine. The more mineral loss, the greater the risk for osteoporosis, osteoarthritis, hypothyroidism, coronary artery disease, high blood pressure, bone spurs, muscle spasms and other degenerative diseases.

"Susan, a nurse, is very overweight. During a visit to my office, she told me she has muscle cramps in her calves that wake her up every night. Being a nurse, she is very health conscious. She read an article in a health magazine that said these kinds of cramps are caused by a lack of potassium or magnesium, so she began eating a banana every night before bedtime. This did not improve her condition at all. After I reviewed her diet, and found out that she often drank highly acidic Diet Coke after her midnight shift. I told her to stop eating bananas and stop drinking soda. I suggested if she felt hungry, she should drink fresh vegetable juice or puree. She later happily reported that all the leg cramps were completely gone in two days and she does not feel sugar cravings or a desire for soft drinks anymore. Her roommate was very surprised she could even refuse offers of soda and chocolate after each night shift. Even amazingly, she started to lose weight. She lost 15 pounds in three weeks."

—DR. PING

Acid waste products are also deposited into fat, organs, tissues and joints causing many sub-health conditions. We now sometimes see sufferers of osteoarthritis as young as 15.

In summary, in order to maintain a healthy body alkaline reserve, we need to eat a predominantly alkaline-forming diet. Another effective way to help increase alkaline reserve is to use a top quality alkaline water, which we'll discuss in Section 2.7.

2.4   NUTRITIONALLY DENSE FOODS

The need to eat a nutritionally dense, low calorie diet is evident. In our automobile analogy, for the car to be "healthy" and last for a long time, not only we need an efficient engine that, when burning gas, leaves as few waste product as possible inside the car, we also need a really high quality clean gas. Low-grade gas yields fewer miles per gallon and leaves the engine dirty.

In the PingLongevity™ Diet, when studying the nutritional value of foods, we mainly look at the food's caloric efficiency. For every calorie we consume, we need to look at the percentage that comes from protein, good fats and good carbohydrates, as well as essential vitamins and minerals. We want less dietary cholesterol per calorie intake.

This is a very unique approach, because most food studies compare foods of the same weight, for example, one gram of rice compared to one gram of nuts. But this is wrong because they contain very different calorie counts! Eating 720 calories can mean you'll get one fat-free, sugar-free muffin or the combination of a whole pineapple, $1/2$ cantaloupe, $1/2$ kiwifruit, $1/2$ papaya, 5 ounces of grapes, 2 pears and 2 whole wheat rolls. Therefore, what we want is to take in substantially fewer calories, while at the same time, consuming much more nutritionally dense foods.

Beginning on page 56 is a detailed PingLongevity™ Diet Basic Food Nutritional Density Comparison Chart.

From the chart, we can draw the following conclusions:

- For grains, flaxseeds, chia, wheat germ, quinoa, oats and amaranth provide the most protein and good fats (unsaturated fats such as omega-3). There are no dietary cholesterols in grains. These are the grains we promote in the PingLongevity™ Diet in place of common grains such as rice and wheat.

- Generally, meat has the highest saturated fat, and cholesterol, even when we choose the leanest meats, but meat is also highest in proteins. The PingLongevity™ Diet requires eating no more than two meat meals per week.

- Eggs are not efficient because they have very high cholesterol, fat content and relatively low proteins compared with meat. However, egg white is a pure protein source without fat or cholesterol.

- Generally, fish is a better protein and fatty acid source than red meat. Seafood including cod, halibut, mahi mahi, monkfish, octopus, orange roughy, pollock, rockfish and scallops are the best fish, high in proteins without saturated fat. Most other fish and seafood is also a better source of proteins and fatty acids than meat. Care must be taken eating shrimp and calamari because of high cholesterol.

- Dairy products, such as milk, yogurt, cheese and ice cream, are generally are high in saturated fat. Therefore, except for nonfat raw milk, the PingLongevity™ Diet does not recommend dairy products unless they are raw, organic and fat free.

- Nuts are good source of monounsaturated fats. Eating nuts in moderation, especially raw soaked nuts, is healthy.

2.4.1   Nutritionally Dense Fat

Body fat provides your most important reservoir of stored energy as adipose tissue. Even in a person who is not overweight, body fat still makes up about 10 percent of body weight. From a survival standpoint, this is absolutely critical, since in periods of low food availability or during a famine situation, a person must live from stored body fat or die. Body fat is also used as a median for the transport of fat-soluble vitamins such as vitamins A, D and K.

Let's examine different kinds of fats we frequently encounter on our plates:

Trans fat is the common name for unsaturated fat with *trans-*isomer fatty acid(s). It may occur naturally in small amounts in animal products.

The other kind of trans-fat is artificially produced by adding hydrogen to liquid oils so they remain solid at room temperature, which helps extend a food's shelf life. Conclusive studies have shown the artificial trans-fat raises levels of LDL ("bad") cholesterol and lowers HDL ("good") cholesterol, raising the risk of heart disease.

Most commercially produced fried foods, baked goods and stick margarines are made with artificial trans fat. Labels may call it hydrogenated vegetable oil. Natural trans fat can be found in red meat, milk, butter and cheese.

Trans fat needs to be avoided as much as possible. Many cities,

GRAINS NUTRITIONAL VALUE

¹/₄ CUP DRY	CALORIES	TOTAL FAT (G)	SATURATED FAT (G)	CHOLESTEROL (MG)	PROTEIN (G)	SODIUM (MG)	CARBOHYDRATE (G)
Amaranth	182	3.25	0.75	0	7	10.25	32.25
Barley	163	1	0.25	0	5.75	5.5	33.75
Buckwheat	146	1.5	0.25	0	5.75	0.5	30.5
Corn	152	2	0.25	0	4	14.5	30.75
Flaxseed	224	17.75	1.5	0	7.75	12.5	12.25
Millet	189	2	0.25	0	5.5	2.5	36.5
Oats	152	2.75	0.5	0	6.5	0.75	25.75
Quinoa	159	2.5	0.25	0	5.5	9	29.25
Rice	171	1.25	0.25	0	3.75	3.25	35.75
Rye	142	1	0	0	6.25	2.5	29.5
Sorghum	163	1.5	0.25	0	5.5	3	33.75
Spelt	140	1	0.25	0	6	0	31
Teff	160	1	0	0	6	10	33
Triticale	161	1	0.25	0	6.25	2.5	34.5
Wheat	158	1	0.25	0	7.5	1	32.75
Wild Rice	143	0.5	0	0	6	2.75	30
Chia (1 oz)	137	9	1	0	4	5	12
Wheatgerm (100g)	360	10	2	0	23	12	52

NUTS NUTRITIONAL VALUE

1 OZ	CALORIES	FAT (G)	SATURATED FAT (G)	CHOLESTEROL (MG)	PROTEIN (G)	SODIUM (MG)	CARBOHYDRATE (G)
Pecans	200	20	2	0	3	—	4
Walnuts	200	20	1.5	0	5	—	3
Almonds	170	14	1.5	0	7	—	6
Cashew	170	15	2.5	0	5	—	8
Peanuts (dry roasted)	170	14	2.5	0	7	—	6
Sesame Seeds	158	13	2	0	5	—	7
Pumpkin or Squash Seeds	125	5	1	0	5	—	15

FIBER (G)	SATURATED/ TOTAL FAT	PROTEIN CAL/ TOTAL CAL	CARB CAL/ TOTAL CAL	UNSATURATED FAT CAL/TOTAL CAL	SATURATED FAT CAL/TOTAL CAL	CHOLESTEROL (MG)/TOTAL CAL
4.5	23%	15%	71%	12%	4%	0.00
8	25%	14%	83%	4%	1%	0.00
4.25	17%	16%	84%	8%	2%	0.00
3	13%	11%	81%	10%	1%	0.00
11.5	8%	14%	22%	65%	6%	0.00
4.25	13%	12%	77%	8%	1%	0.00
4.25	18%	17%	68%	13%	3%	0.00
2.5	10%	14%	74%	13%	1%	0.00
1.5	20%	9%	84%	5%	1%	0.00
6.25	0%	18%	83%	6%	0%	0.00
3	17%	13%	83%	7%	1%	0.00
3	25%	17%	89%	5%	2%	0.00
6	0%	15%	83%	6%	0%	0.00
0	25%	16%	86%	4%	1%	0.00
5.75	25%	19%	83%	4%	1%	0.00
2.5	0%	17%	84%	3%	0%	0.00
11	11%	12%	35%	53%	7%	0.00
13	20%	26%	58%	20%	5%	0.00

FIBER (G)	SATURATED/ TOTAL FAT	PROTEIN CAL/ TOTAL CAL	CARB CAL/ TOTAL CAL	UNSATURATED FAT CAL/TOTAL CAL	SATURATED FAT CAL/TOTAL CAL	CHOLESTEROL (MG)/TOTAL CAL
—	10%	6%	8%	81%	9%	0.00
—	8%	10%	6%	83%	7%	0.00
—	11%	16%	14%	66%	8%	0.00
—	17%	12%	19%	66%	13%	0.00
—	18%	16%	14%	61%	13%	0.00
—	15%	13%	18%	63%	11%	0.00
—	20%	16%	48%	29%	7%	0.00

MEAT NUTRITIONAL VALUE

3 OUNCE SERVING SIZE	CALORIES	TOTAL FAT (G)	SATURATED FAT (G)	CHOLESTEROL (MG)	PROTEIN (G)	SODIUM (MG)	CARBOHYDRATE (G)
Lamb Shank	153	5.7	2	74	24	—	—
Lamb Chop (fat trimmed)	180	8	3	80	25	—	—
Beef Tenderloin (fat trimmed, roasted)	180	8.5	3.2	70	24	—	—
Beef Sirloin (fat trimmed)	170	6.1	2.4	75	26	—	—
Ground Beef (90% lean)	210	11	4	85	27	—	—
Pork Tenderloin (fat trimmed, roasted)	139	4.1	1.4	67	26	—	—
Pork Chop (fat trimmed)	170	7	2	70	26	—	—
Chicken Breast (skin on, roasted)	170	7	2	70	25	—	—
Turkey Leg (skin on, roasted)	177	8.3	2.6	72	24	—	—
Turkey Breast (skin on, roasted)	161	6.3	1.8	67	24	—	—
Whole Chicken Egg (1 large)	75	5	1.6	213	6.7	—	—
Egg White (1 large)	17	0	0	0	4	—	—
Egg Yolk (1 large)	58	5	1.6	213	2.7	—	—

DAIRY NUTRITIONAL VALUE

1 CUP FEDERAL STANDARDS	CALORIES	FAT (G)	SATURATED FAT (G)	CHOLESTEROL (MG)	PROTEIN (G)	SODIUM (MG)	CARBOHYDRATE (G)
Nonfat Milk	90	1	1	8	8	—	12
Lowfat 2% Milk	122	5	3	22	8	—	12
Whole Milk	152	8	5	35	8	—	12
Yogurt, Plain Low-Fat	144	4	2.3	14	12	—	16
American Cheese (1oz)	106	8.9	5.6	27	6.3	—	0.5
Cheddar Cheese (1oz)	114	9.4	6	30	7.1	—	0.4
Swiss Cheese (1oz)	107	7.8	5	26	8.1	—	1
Ice Cream, Vanilla ($1/_2$ cup)	132	7.3	4.5	29	2.3	—	15.5
Ice Cream, Low-fat	92	2.8	1.7	9	2.5	—	15

FIBER (G)	SATURATED/ TOTAL FAT	PROTEIN CAL/ TOTAL CAL	CARB CAL/ TOTAL CAL	UNSATURATED FAT CAL/TOTAL CAL	SATURATED FAT CAL/TOTAL CAL	CHOLESTEROL (MG)/TOTAL CAL
—	35%	63%	—	22%	12%	0.48
—	38%	56%	—	25%	15%	0.44
—	38%	53%	—	27%	16%	0.39
—	39%	61%	—	20%	13%	0.44
—	36%	51%	—	30%	17%	0.40
—	34%	75%	—	17%	9%	0.48
—	29%	61%	—	26%	11%	0.41
—	29%	59%	—	26%	11%	0.41
—	31%	54%	—	29%	13%	0.41
—	29%	60%	—	25%	10%	0.42
—	32%	36%	—	41%	19%	2.84
—	N/A	94%	—	0%	0%	0.00
—	32%	19%	—	53%	25%	3.67

FIBER (G)	SATURATED/ TOTAL FAT	PROTEIN CAL/ TOTAL CAL	CARB CAL/ TOTAL CAL	UNSATURATED FAT CAL/TOTAL CAL	SATURATED FAT CAL/TOTAL CAL	CHOLESTEROL (MG)/TOTAL CAL
—	100%	36%	53%	0%	10%	0.09
—	60%	26%	39%	15%	22%	0.18
—	63%	21%	32%	18%	30%	0.23
—	58%	33%	44%	11%	14%	0.10
—	63%	24%	2%	28%	48%	0.25
—	64%	25%	1%	27%	47%	0.26
—	64%	30%	4%	24%	42%	0.24
—	62%	7%	47%	19%	31%	0.22
—	61%	11%	65%	11%	17%	0.10

FISH NUTRITIONAL VALUE

1 CUP FEDERAL STANDARDS	CALORIES	FAT (G)	SATURATED FAT (G)	CHOLESTEROL (MG)	PROTEIN (G)	SODIUM (MG)	CARBOHYDRATE (G)
Calamari (4 oz/raw)	80	2.5	1.5	215	15	—	—
Catfish	140	9	2	50	17	—	—
Cod	90	0.5	0	45	20	—	—
Rainbow Trout	140	6	2	60	21	—	—
Halibut	110	2	0	35	23	—	—
Mackerel	210	13	1.5	60	21	—	—
Mahi Mahi	90	0.75	0	60	19.5	—	—
Monkfish	82	2	0	27	16	—	—
Octopus	70	1	0	20	16	—	—
Orange Roughy	80	1	0	20	16	—	—
Pollock	90	1	0	80	20	—	—
Rockfish	100	2	0	40	21	—	—
Scallops (14 small/6 large)	120	1	0	55	22	—	—
Salmon/Atlantic	160	7	1	59	22	—	—
Salmon/Sockeye	180	9	1.5	75	23	—	—
Salmon/King	200	12	3	70	21	—	—
Salmon/chum/ Pink	130	4	1	70	22	—	—
Smoked Salmon (2oz)	140	9	3	35	11	—	-
Sole	100	1.5	0.5	60	21	—	—
Striped Bass (3/5 oz raw)	100	1.5	0.5	80	18	—	—
Sword Fish	130	4.5	1	40	22	—	—
Tilapia	110	2.5	1	75	22	—	—
Tuna/Yellow-Fin	150	4	0	49	20	—	—
Shrimp (3oz boiled)	110	2	0	160	22	—	—
Oyster, steamed, 12 medium	120	4	1	90	12	—	—

Fiber (G)	Saturated/ Total Fat	Protein cal/ Total Cal	Carb cal/ Total Cal	Unsaturated Fat cal/Total Cal	Saturated Fat Cal/Total Cal	Cholesterol (mg)/Total Cal
—	60%	75%	—	11%	17%	2.69
—	22%	49%	—	45%	13%	0.36
—	0%	89%	—	5%	0%	0.50
—	33%	60%	—	26%	13%	0.43
—	0%	84%	—	16%	0%	0.32
—	12%	40%	—	49%	6%	0.29
—	0%	87%	—	8%	0%	0.67
—	0%	78%	—	22%	0%	0.33
—	0%	91%	—	13%	0%	0.29
—	0%	80%	—	11%	0%	0.25
—	0%	89%	—	10%	0%	0.89
—	0%	84%	—	18%	0%	0.40
—	0%	73%	—	8%	0%	0.46
—	14%	55%	—	34%	6%	0.37
—	17%	51%	—	38%	8%	0.42
—	25%	42%	—	41%	14%	0.35
—	25%	68%	—	21%	7%	0.54
—	33%	31%	—	39%	19%	0.25
—	33%	84%	—	9%	5%	0.60
—	33%	72%	—	9%	5%	0.80
—	22%	68%	—	24%	7%	0.31
—	40%	80%	—	12%	8%	0.68
—	0%	53%	—	24%	0%	0.33
—	0%	80%	—	16%	0%	1.45
—	25%	40%	—	23%	8%	0.75

including New York, Los Angeles, Philadelphia and Boston have legislation pending to limit or ban artificial trans fat in foods sold in restaurants. A product must contain less than 0.5 grams of trans fat per serving in order to bear a "no trans fat" label, according to the Food and Drug Administration.

Saturated fat, another bad fat, is fat that consists of triglycerides containing only saturated fatty acid radicals, which raises LDL cholesterol and sets the stage for heart disease by encouraging the formation of plaque in arteries.

> " 'Just one meal high in saturated fat may damage blood vessels and hinder the ability of HDL cholesterol to protect arteries. Normally, HDL guards blood vessels from inflammation that contributes to artery-clogging plaque,' says Stephen Nicholls, M.D., a cardiologist at the Cleveland Clinic Foundation.
>
> Not so after a meal high in saturated fat. When Nicholls and colleagues fed 14 healthy volunteers two meals of carrot cake and a milk shake-one made with highly saturated coconut oil and one with polyunsaturated safflower oil-two things happened: The ability of blood vessels to expand and contract (a sign of healthy arteries) and the anti-inflammatory action of HDL were impaired for as much as six hours after the high saturated fat meal. In contrast, when the cake and milk shake were made with polyunsaturated fat, arterial and HDL functions improved. Just how much saturated fat was in that test meal?
>
> 'We likened it to people eating a double cheeseburger, fries and a shake, which, unfortunately, is not that uncommon a meal,' Nicholls says."
>
> —*CNN NEWS,* JULY 22, 2008

Saturated fat should be avoided as much as possible. It is found mostly in animal products such as whole milk, cream, butter, lard and red meats. It is also found in cocoa butter and tropical palm, palm kernel and coconut oils.

Monounsaturated fat has a single double bond in the fatty acid chain and all of the remainder of the carbon atoms in the chain are single-bonded. Monounsaturated fat helps lower blood cholesterol levels when substituted for saturated fat in the diet. It is found mostly in olives and avocados and olive, canola and peanut oils. We should use monounsaturated fats as substitutes for all trans fat and saturated fats.

Polyunsaturated fat is a fatty acid in which more than one double bond exists within the representative molecule. This type of fat helps reduce blood cholesterol levels when substituted for saturated fats. It is found mostly in nuts, cheese, seeds, fish, krill, algae, leafy greens and safflower, sunflower, sesame, corn and soy oils.

Omega-3 fatty acids, a type of polyunsaturated fat, are particularly healthy. They include α-linolenic acid (ALA), eicosapentaenoic acid (EPA) and docosahexaenoic acid (DHA). Omega-3 fatty acids can be found in fatty fish such as salmon and mackerel, flaxseed, chia seeds and walnuts. Studies have shown significant health benefits from lowering blood pressure, controlling inflammation, preventing blood platelets from clumping together, protecting against irregular heartbeats, increasing retina and brain function and reducing tumor growth.

Two studies from the University of Pittsburgh suggest omega-3s found in fish may help improve mood and increase gray matter in the brain. In the first, researchers demonstrated that people with high blood levels of omega-3s tended to be more agreeable and less likely to report mild symptoms of depression than those with low levels. In the second study, researchers uncovered a possible mechanism behind the mood differences: People with high blood levels of omega-3s have more gray matter in the areas of the brain linked to mood. Although preliminary, the findings provide increasing support for including omega-3s in a healthful diet.

In one study, two groups of pigs were fed an unhealthy diet, high in cholesterol, sugar and fat. But one group had an added high dosage of omega-3 fish oil. Both groups have similar poor readings for LDL cholesterol and triglycerides. But six months later, it was discovered that the blood vessels of the pigs fed omega-3 were clear, while the other group had extensive cholesterol deposits on the arterial walls.

In cooking, the worst fats are: butter, cocoa butter, coconut oil, lard, margarine (hard), palm oil and palm kernel oil. The best polyunsaturated oils are: mustard, canola, almond, macadamia nut, olive, soybean and flaxseed. An added benefit of canola, soybean and flaxseed oils is that they are high in omega-3 fatty acids.

In summary, you should avoid trans fat and saturated fat. This means to avoid all fats from red meat animals, including full-fat dairy products. If you eat meat, choose extra lean cuts. Use non-fat dairy products. Replace your oils as much as possible with omega-3 oils, using them in salad dressings. Eat foods rich in omega-3s and take fish oil supplements.

2.4.2   Nutritionally Dense Proteins

Proteins (also known as polypeptides) are organic compounds made of amino acids arranged in a linear chain and folded into a globular form. Animals (including humans) must obtain some of the amino acids from their diets. Amino acids that an organism cannot synthesize on its own are referred to as essential amino acids.

For humans, essential amino acids include isoleucine, leucine, lysine, methionine, phenylalanine, threonine, tryptophan, valine, histidine, tyrosine and selenocysteine. Non-essential amino acids include alanine, arginine, aspartate, cysteine, glutamate, glutamine, glycine, proline, serine, asparagine and pyrrolysine.

Proteins are very important molecules in our cells. They are involved in virtually all cell functions. There are many different type of proteins, including antibodies for defending us from antigens, contractile proteins for muscle building, hormonal proteins for delivering the body's control messages, structural proteins for building connective tissues, storage proteins for storing amino acids and transport proteins as carriers for hemoglobin and cytochromes in the blood.

A complete protein consists of not only all essential amino acids, but it must also be in proper proportions. Generally, proteins derived from animal foods (meats, fish, poultry, cheese, eggs, yogurt and milk) are complete. Proteins derived from plant foods (legumes, grains and vegetables) tend to be partial in essential amino acids.

However, there are non-meat sources of complete proteins, including egg whites, soy protein isolate, amaranth, aphanizomenon flos-aquae (a type of blue-green algae), buckwheat, hempseed, soybeans, quinoa, chia and spirulina.

In his book, *The China Study,* Dr. Colin Campbell eloquently presented extensive scientific data demonstrating that animal protein has a direct causal relationship to degenerative diseases.

Dr. Ganmaa Davaasambuu, a Harvard researcher noted that ingestion of natural estrogens in cows' milk may be linked to breast, prostate and testicular cancers in humans. All of these cancers are "hormone-dependent" tumors, meaning that they need sex hormones to grow. He cited a study comparing diet and cancer rates in 42 countries that showed a strong correlation between milk and cheese consumption and the incidence of testicular cancer among men ages 20 to 39, increased death rates from prostate cancer and breast cancer.

As a result of all these animal protein studies, we should try to minimize our intake of animal (except for fish) proteins. Instead, we should use multiple plant-based protein sources in order to comprise a complete protein diet.

2.4.3 Nutritionally Dense Carbohydrates

A carbohydrate is an organic compound with the empirical formula $C_m(H_2O)_n$, that consists only of carbon, hydrogen and oxygen, with the last two in the 2:1 atom ratio. The simplest carbohydrates are called monosaccharides, which include glucose, fructose and sucrose. It's basically simple sugar. Monosaccharides are the major source of fuel for metabolism, being used both as an energy source (glucose being the most important in nature) and in biosynthesis. When many cells do not immediately need monosaccharides, they are often converted to more space efficient forms, often polysaccharides. In many animals, including humans, this storage form is glycogen, especially in liver and muscle cells.

The body needs both nutrition and energy. For energy, the body can use carbohydrates more efficiently than fat and proteins, as discussed in Section 2.2.3. Therefore, a good balanced diet must contain carbohydrates.

There's nothing more confusing than carbohydrates. The world is full of scientific studies, expert advice and fad diets, all telling you different things, some low-carb, others a certain percent of carb in your food, yet others wanting you to eat a pure carb vegan diet. Which one is correct?

For example, in 2008, the Atkins Foundation funded a comprehensive study, led by Harvard Professor Meir Stampfer. The research was done in a controlled environment—an isolated nuclear research facility in Israel. The 322 participants got lunch, their main meal of the day, a central cafeteria. The result shows that the low-carb diet helped people lose more weight than a traditional low-fat diet in one of the longest and largest studies to compare the dueling weight-loss techniques.

The Mayo Clinic diet requires you to eat 45–65% carbohydrates, while the Atkins diet is totally against carbohydrates.

> "I ran into a well-known nutritionist and body builder, who frequently appears in newspapers and magazines and on TV shows. He told me about his diet discovery that involved total avoidance of carbohydrates. He decided he'd make it a new diet.
>
> 'Wait, let's not create another fad diet,' I thought as we talked.
>
> I wondered why not a single "expert" talks about THE WAY carbohydrates are processed and cooked. Don't people know that the reason carbohydrates got such a bad name is that processing and refining foods, as well as cooking, have reduced complex wholesome carbohydrates into refined simple carbohydrates? That's why I always tell people, when you eat a bowl of rice or a slice of bread, in fact you're eating pure sugar!"
>
> —DR. PING

It's apparent that many of these scientific studies and expert advice are biased because there's no mention of the way food is processed and cooked.

When in raw and whole food form, carbohydrates are complex, and naturally have a low glycemic index. They do not tend to increase weight when the total calorie intake is proper.

There are low starch and high starch carbohydrates. These can easily be distinguished when cooking. For example, if you cook a rice-based soup until it is very well done, you'll find the soup to be very starchy. This is a result of heat breaking down the granules and freeing up individual molecules. On the other hand, if you do the same thing with quinoa, a South American grain, no matter how much you cook it, you won't get a starchy, sticky soup.

Therefore, we must classify carbohydrates into high-starch carb and low-starch carb. We must also distinguish between raw, refined and cooked, simple and complex. The best diet should have a good amount of whole, raw low-starch carbohydrates.

Good carbohydrates include: vegetables and fruits, certain grains such as flaxseed, wheat germ, chia seed, quinoa, black sesame, hempseed, sweet potato and corn.

In the PingLongevity™ Diet, we eat a balanced diet with a good proportion of *raw* carbohydrates. For example, if you soak a few of teaspoons of chia seeds in raw fat-free milk for 10 minutes, you'll find that it becomes soft and delicious to eat. You might also try to eat sweet potatoes or corn raw.

2.4.4   Farmed and Genetically Engineered Foods

Fundamentally, we are not against lean red meat. Beef and lamb, for example, have high nutritional value. After all, some of the pure meat eaters, such as the Masai, Eskimo and Mongolians are healthy and do not experience degenerative diseases in their traditional settings.

The problem may lie with modern technology: farmed and genetically engineered animals. Because of this, we advise you to avoid eating farmed raised non-organic animal meat and dairy products.

Dr. Ganmaa Davaasambuu of Harvard University believes that natural estrogens are 100,000 times more potent than environmental estrogens and that today's cow's milk is particularly rich in them.

The reason is that dairy farmers now milk their cows about 300 days per year. For much of that time, the cows are pregnant and as pregnancy progresses, the estrogen content of their milk increases. This causes hormone related cancers such as breast, ovarian, prostate and testicular cancer.

Another of Dr. Davaasambuu's studies showed increased hormone levels among Mongolian third-graders after a month of drinking commercial milk from the United States.

According to a 2008 sampling survey of farmed fish, tilapia (the fastest growing and most widely farmed fish) and catfish have much lower concentrations of omega-3s, very high ratios of omega-6 to omega-3, and high saturated and mono-unsaturated fat to omega-3 ratios. The study's authors noted that "marked changes in the fishing industry during the past decade have produced widely eaten fish that have fatty acid characteristics that are generally accepted to be inflammatory by the health care community."

In 2007, according to a study conducted by researchers from the Louis Bolk Institute in the Netherlands, young children who exclusively consume organic dairy products are significantly less likely to develop allergies, asthma or eczema by the age of two.

Another modern miracle is how we farm. Nowadays, everything—apples, corn, watermelon—looks bigger and prettier, but has less taste. Animals—chicken, fish, pigs, cows, sheep—all grow bigger and faster. Milking cows become more productive. This is a result of lots genetic engineering and modifying, chemicals and fertilizers, hormones and antibiotics. It's very difficult for us to avoid such foods. They are everywhere!

To try to minimize the negative impact of farmed food, we should eat as little inorganic red meat and farmed fish as possible. Additionally, if possible, eat only organic fruits and vegetables.

2.4.5   High Temperature Cooked Foods

High temperature has a significant impact on fat, protein and carbohydrates.

Cooking at high temperatures can damage fat. The more omega-

3 fatty acids are the present in the oil, the less suitable it is for cooking. The heat not only damages the fatty acids, it can also change them into harmful substances. Hydrogenated oils (trans fat) are often used for cooking because these oils have already been "damaged" by chemical processing, they are less likely to be further damaged by heat. The oils that are higher in saturated fats or monounsaturates are the most stable when heated. Sizzling fat on a grill generates cancer-causing substances such as nitrosamines, hydrocarbons and benzopyrene.

Overcooking creates chemical changes that can alter or destroy protein. Excess heat breaks down proteins, causing them to lose essential amino acids and up to 50 percent of their vitamins and minerals. Also, the higher the temperature, the more cancer-causing chemicals are produced. Meat, fish and poultry cooked on a gas grill create nitrosamines, which are carcinogens. When meat is charred, polycyclic hydrocarbons and free radicals are created.

As discussed in Section 2.4.3, heat can break down carbohydrates from complex to simple, making them essentially very similar to pure sugar in structure.

Therefore, we should avoid high temperature cooking and high temperature processed foods. Nuts, the type widely sold commercially, require particular attention because in order to be tasty, they usually are processed at high temperatures. How do you tell? If the nuts are very crispy, they are very likely to have been high temp processed. If you just put raw nuts into your home oven at the usual baking temperature, you'll produce a roasted nut that is not so crispy.

2.4.6   Empty Calorie Foods

Empty calorie foods are those that have little nutritional value. At the top if this list are pure sugar and refined flour. This includes cakes, pies, pastries, candy and soft drinks. Empty calories are also found in unhealthy fats in fried foods such as French fries, stir fried dishes, fried seafood and chicken.

Artificial sweeteners (sugar alcohols) should also be avoided. Foods that contain sugar alcohols can be labeled sugar-free because they replace full calorie sugar sweeteners. Sugar provides 4 kcal/gram and sugar alcohols provide an average of 2 kcal/gram. The bottom line is that even at half of the calories, sweeteners retain the same properties as sugar, i.e., empty calories and high glycemic index. There's an added problem: Recent research conducted at UCSD in an article entitled "Artificial Sweeteners Confound the Brain; May Lead to Diet Disaster," showed that Splenda is not satisfying—at least according to the brain. A new study found that even when the palate cannot distinguish between the artificial sweetener and sugar, the brain knows the difference. If that theory plays out, there could be implications for those who use artificial sweeteners as a weight-control aid. Recent research indeed suggests a correlation between artificial sweetener intake and compromised health. In one large survey, diet soda consumption was found to be associated with elevated cardiovascular and metabolic disease risk.

A different study reveals a possible mechanism behind this effect: Rats fed artificially sweetened yogurt in addition to their regular feed ended up eating more and gaining more weight than rats fed yogurt with real sugar.

Many experts advocate eating chocolate for the flavonols in cocoa. It was recently reported by Brian Buijsse of the German Institute of Human Nutrition in Nuthetal, Germany, published in the *European Heart Journal* that consuming 7.5 grams of chocolate daily resulted in significantly lower blood pressure than consuming just a sprinkle of it daily. While we agree with the benefit of cocoa, we are concerned about the amount of sugar in most of the chocolates on the market. We advise our patients to eat extra dark (>70% cocoa) chocolates to reduce the side effect of empty calories.

If you really require sweet flavors in cooking, for example in making your own salad dressing, it's better to use raw honey than sugar. This is because honey contains at least 15 nutrients, whereas sugar has none. Honey is an aid to digestion when taken in the raw state due to its enzyme content, while sugar interferes with digestion. Honey enters the bloodstream slowly, at a rate of two calories per minute, while sugar enters quickly at 10 calories per minute, causing blood sugars to fluctuate rapidly and wildly. Sugar is highly acidic causing calcium leakage from bones, contributing to osteoporosis while honey does not. You may also choose papaya and pineapple to spice up your food flavor.

Pasteurized fruit juice should be avoided. Due to a lack of food enzymes, it resembles sugary water. Make your own raw fresh squeezed fruit juice, or if you have to buy juice, make sure it is completely unprocessed!

Alcohol lovers like the studies that show red wine is good for cardiovascular function and a good source of antioxidants. While it's true that red grapes and grape seeds are highly nutritious, wine of course contains alcohol, which is not only high in calories, but also an oxidant. In general, alcohol is high in calories, but low in nutrition.

2.4.7   Longevity Herbs

There are several herbs traditionally known to be overall life extenders. They should be integrated in your diet. For example, we have them in the PingLongevity™ Mix, as discussed at the beginning of this chapter.

- **He Shou Wu:** The ancient story said that there was an old fellow living in a small village. He could not get married because he was impotent, weak and very poor. At age 54, he had a dream about taking a kind of grass root he'd seen high up in the mountains to restore his sexual vitality and transmute this newfound energy into long life. When he woke up, he went to fetch this root. After taking the herb, his hair turned from gray back to black. His cheeks and lips turned red and opaque, full of vibrant light. He restored his sexual vitality. He was stronger than ever. He got married at age 59, had six children, and died at age 160.

- **Goji Berry (Wolfberry):** It's one of the most powerful anti-aging foods. It is nutritionally rich, containing beta-carotene, vitamins C, B1, B2, B6, E and other vitamins, minerals, antioxidants, and amino acids, isoleucine, tryptophan, zinc, iron, copper, calcium, germanium, selenium and phosphorus. In TCM, it is believed to enhance immune system function, help eyesight, protect the liver, boost sperm production, improve circulation, balance the liver, lung and kidney channels and enrich yin energy.

- **Ginseng:** It is the widely recognized and used in TCM. Ginseng is believed to boost the body's vital essence and chi, calm the spirit, and enhance body's immune system. American Ginseng is mild and suitable as a food supplement.

- **Astragalus:** Astragalus has been used in TCM for thousands of years. It helps protect the body against various stresses, including physical, mental and emotional stress. It contains antioxidants, which protect cells against damage caused by free radicals, byproducts of cellular energy. Astragalus is used to protect and support the immune system, for preventing colds and upper respiratory infections, to lower blood pressure, to treat diabetes and to protect the liver.

2.5   FOOD ORDER AND COMBINING

Many people like to eat fruit at the end of a meal. In the East, people also drink soup at the end of a meal. Neither one is a good idea. If you eat fruit with meal, you should always eat it first. This is because fruit digestion mostly occurs in the small intestine rather than in the stomach. You don't want fruit mixed up with other foods in the stomach where it will dilute stomach acid.

Soup or other liquids should follow the fruit also to avoid diluting stomach acid.

Eat your main protein and carbohydrates last.

2.6   THE NEW HEALTH FOOD INDUSTRY

Last year, we visited several "whole food" and "health food" markets. We also stopped by Natural Products Expo West, where thousands of "whole" and "health" food manufacturers exhibit. For completeness, we also took a look at the shelves in the stores of large fitness centers.

While we applaud the movement that seems to be moving towards more "organic" and "whole" foods, we have to caution our patients of inherent issues of the approach.

Here is our main observation: In general, if you go to a normal supermarket, take the processed foods, replace the ingredients with "organic" ones, you get the "healthy foods" that are being marketed by this new movement.

We'll tell you the problem in a few examples.

Example 1.

Let's take a look at this "healthy food" eatery within a "health food" store. If everything is "organic" and "whole", is it OK to eat oil-based salad dressings, high starch buns, deep fried meat and super sweet chocolate cakes?

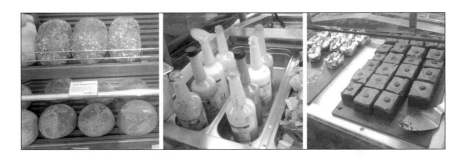

For the PingLongevity™ Diet, we use raw ingredients (such as lime, miso, papaya, pineapple, chili pepper) without oil for salad dressing; we eat low-starch, nutrient rich grains in their raw form (quinoa, chia, flaxseeds, wheat germ, sweet potatoes); wild small ocean fish in place of meat and healthy desserts in place of sweets.

Example 2.

It appears that everyone is coming up with some kind of expensive drinks, exotic fruit drinks, energy drinks, vegetable drinks and all kinds of special waters. We have even seen "quinoa drinks." We stopped by the booth advertising this vegetable drink as "wild, wholesome, all-natural, America's next food."

We dug into how it is made. We were told, "It's heated just below the boiling point to preserve the wholeness." Well, you are talking about 212 degrees Fahrenheit! Tell me that this drink is still nutritious as the raw vegetable juice? Recall that food enzymes are destroyed at 118 degrees F (Section 2.1).

Every time, we stopped by a juice booth, we always asked if the just is pasteurized. Most are! So you're much better off if you do a little exercise and squeeze or blend your own highly nutritious and cost effective fruit and vegetable juice!

Example 3.

We ran into hundreds of food bars (nutrition, energy, wellness, power, greens, anti-oxidants, etc.). We don't want to put up pictures here because making enemies is not our purpose.

But let us analyze a label. This is an energy bar, with a total calorie count of 145, of which 31% comes from saturated fat and 30% from sugar! OK, We do agree that beside the 61% bad calories, you got some other stuff, proteins, egg, white wheat flour, honey, vanilla, baking soda, salt and cholesterol.

Do you still think you are eating "healthy energy" foods?

Example 4.

We have many examples but we don't want to make this section too long. We'll end with a funny one :-) —the organic cheeseburger!

2.7   LONGEVITY, WATER AND AIR

We cannot talk about a healthy diet without discussing water and air. After all, water and air are not only in every part of our bodies, but they are also a subtle energy source.

Both water and air are important carriers of energy. For example, a homeopathic pill is made by dissolving herbs into water and diluting the solution until no herbal molecules remain. The resulting homeopathic remedy contains only water molecules without any chemical trace of herbs. How, then, is the remedy effective?

The water is actually modulated to the herbs' vibrational frequencies. If the herbs are tuned to the frequency of the energy centers of the body, (a topic we will take up later in chapter 10), using the modulated water would potentially help heal the body.

Similarly, some chi-gong masters use their hands to emit chi into water and then send the water to patients for remote healing. Very high-energy water, such as spring water directly from high mountains, absorbs a lot of cosmic energy. The more spiritually developed you are (and thereby more attuned to higher frequencies), the more you are able to absorb energy from high-energy water.

Air is another important energy source. High-energy air is air that is charged with negative ions and cosmic energy. The negative ions are now measurable by modern instruments; cosmic energy is yet to be measured.

Industrialization has eliminated most high-energy water and air from our environment. Water is polluted, treated and re-circulated. California recently passed a resolution to re-claim bathroom water for drinking water. In large office buildings, shopping malls and factories, air is de-ionized through filters and air conditioning. Fresh air is neutralized through windows with metal frames and screens. Dead air is re-circulated over and over again. Smog from traffic and industrial pollution also neutralizes the air. Not only does pollution poison the body, but this dead air carries little higher energy.

We talk about getting "re-charged" when we spend time by the ocean or in the mountains. Ocean or mountain breezes make you feel "charged" because of the high energy of the air, which contains large amounts of negative ions. Polluted air has clusters with positive electricity, which neutralize the negative ions. Negative ions increase our energy levels and help cleanse the body. In fact, studies show that the human body resembles a semiconductor, which conducts electricity under certain conditions. Air that is high in negative ions literally charges the body.

Oxygen is a major component of high-energy air. When there is a high percentage of oxygen in the air, the body is required to perform less work and our respiratory processes are therefore more efficient. Over the course of a lifetime, this efficiency makes a huge difference in terms of longevity.

Thus, the energy in air depends on the level of negative ionization, the percentage of oxygen, the percentage of pollutants and the percentage of higher energies it carries. The more time we spend in an environment that has pure, high-energy air and water, the more higher energy we can absorb into our bodies.

2.7.1   Ionized Alkaline Water

We rank water from most preferred to least in the following order:

1. High quality ionized alkaline water

2. High quality natural spring water

3. Purified water

4. Distilled water

5. Boiled tap water

Almost 99% time, we only drink the top two kinds. How important is water? When you drink water, within 30 seconds it gets into your blood; within 60 seconds it gets to your brain and reproductive organs; within 30 minutes, it gets to all parts of your body. Our body is about 60–70% water in weight, therefore, make sure you drink the healthiest water.

A good alkaline water ionizer and purifier have the following properties:

• Filter out pollutants, such as chlorine, heavy metals such as arsenic, copper, iron, lead, volatile organic compounds such as pesticides and herbicides, fluoride, bacteria, and pharmaceutical drugs.

• Produce water with pH higher than 9: When water has electrical energy, it causes the hydrogen within it to assume one of two forms. One is hydrogen that has a positive electrical charge H+. This water is "acidic." The other is hydrogen that bonds with an oxygen atom and becomes negatively charged. This is the building block of life itself, and chemically, it is in the form of OH–. Note that this is very different from "hard" water, which also has higher pH. "Hard" water is due to a higher concentration of alkaline minerals. In comparison, tap water has a pH 6–8.5.

- Produce negative ions: In tap water that feeds into the ionizer, there are many mineral molecules, such as calcium, magnesium and potassium. The ionizer produces water with negatively charged (alkaline) minerals.

- Increased oxygen: As ionized alkaline water contain vast number of OH–, it doubles oxygen contents.

- Have an ORP (oxidation reduction potential) more negative than –300mv: ORP measures the electrical charge of water. When it is negative, the water acts as a powerful antioxidant. ORP of most U.S. tab water is between +300~600mv. Most bottled water has ORP above +400mv.

- Have much better hydrating property: Water molecules like to cluster themselves. Ionizers reduce water clusters to hexagonal or smaller, making it easier for the water molecules to enter cells.

> "Recently, I had a whole family who came into the clinic with various complaints. The wife had severe muscle cramps and aching hips. She wakes up every night and has to massage her hips for over an hour. The daughter had severe eczema. Among other things, I asked them to switch from drinking reverse osmosis water, which has no minerals and is acidic, to ionized alkaline water. After drinking alkaline water, within 10 days the mother's pain disappeared, and the daughter's eczema improved."
>
> —DR. PING

There is controversy concerning the effect of alkaline water in the body.

Some well-known scientists and scholars argue that since the stomach is highly acidic, any alkaline water will be neutralized as soon as it enters. To answer this, the following is a quote from the famous U.S. biochemist, Dr. Sang Whang:

"Among the people who question the validity of alkaline water, the biggest question is, 'What happens to the alkaline water once it reaches the stomach, which is highly acidic?' People who have some knowledge of the human body, including medical doctors, ask this question.

Let me answer that question once and for all to erase any doubts about the health benefits of alkaline water.

In order to digest food and kill the kinds of bacteria and viruses that come with food, the inside of our stomach is acidic. The stomach pH level is maintained at around 4. When we eat food and drink water, especially alkaline water, the pH level inside the stomach goes up. When this happens, there is a feed-back mechanism in our stomach to detect this that commands the stomach wall to secrete more hydrochloric acid into the stomach to bring the pH level back to 4. So the stomach becomes acidic again. When we drink more alkaline water, more hydrochloric acid is secreted to maintain the stomach pH value. It seems like a losing battle.

However, when you understand how the stomach wall makes hydrochloric acid, your concerns will disappear. As pathologists explain, there is no hydrochloric acid pouch in our bodies. If there were, it would burn a hole in the body. The cells in the stomach wall must produce it on an instantly-as-needed basis. The ingredients in the stomach cell that make hydrochloric acid (HCl) are carbon dioxide (CO_2), water (H_2O), and sodium chloride (NaCl) or potassium chloride (KCl). $NaCl + H_2O + CO_2 = HCl + NaHCO_3$, or $KCl + H_2O + CO_2 = HCl + KHCO_3$.

As we can see, the byproduct of making hydrochloric acid is sodium bicarbonate ($NaHCO_3$) or potassium bicarbonate ($KHCO_3$), which goes into the bloodstream. These bicarbon-ates are the alkaline buffers that neutralize excess acids in the blood; they dissolve solid acid wastes into liquid form. As they neutralize the solid acidic wastes, extra carbon dioxide is released, which is discharged through the lungs. As the body ages, these alkaline buffers diminish. This phenomenon is called acidosis, a natural occurrence as the body accumulates more acidic waste products. There is, therefore, a relationship between the aging process and the accumulation of acids.

By looking at the pH value of the stomach alone, it seems that alkaline water never reaches the body. But when you look at the whole body, there is a net gain of alkalinity as we drink alkaline water. All cells are slightly alkaline. In order for them to produce acid, they must also produce alkaline and vice versa, just as a water ionizer cannot produce alkaline water without producing acid water, since tap water is almost neutral.

When the stomach pH value gets higher than 4, the stomach can automatically lower the alkalinity. However, if the pH value goes below 4, for any reason, the stomach can't cope with the excess acidity. That's why we take Alka-Seltzer, which is alkaline, to relieve the gas and pain caused by excessive stomach acid. In this case, the stomach wall does not produce hydrochloric acid, therefore, no alkaline buffer is being added to the bloodstream.

The pancreas also produces acid in order to produce alkaline. After the food in the stomach is digested, it moves into the small intestine. The food at this point is so acidic that it will damage the intestine wall. In order to avoid this problem, the pancreas makes alkaline substances (known as pancreatic juice). This juice is essentially sodium bicarbonate and it is mixed with the acidic partially digested food leaving the stomach. From the above formula, in order to produce bicarbonates, the pancreas must make hydrochloric acid, which goes into the blood stream.

We often experience sleepiness after a big meal (not during the meal or while the food is being digested in the stomach), when the digested food is leaving the stomach. That's the time when hydrochloric acid goes into our blood. Hydrochloric acid is the main ingredient in antihistamines that causes drowsiness.

"Alkaline or acid produced by the body must have equal and opposite acid or alkaline production; therefore, there is no net gain. However, alkaline supplied from outside the body, like drinking alkaline water, results in a net gain of alkalinity in our bodies."

—DR. SANG WHANG

One caution is that alkaline ionized water generally cannot be bottled because in a few hours, the water will neutralize itself. Therefore, you need to have an access to a high quality machine.

2.7.2   Ionic Air Purifiers

In general, we prefer negative ion air purifiers to other types of air purifiers. This is because ion air purifiers generate energy charged air, similar to that found at ocean beaches, in the mountains and after a rainfall. Other types of filters only clean pollutants out of the air.

A good negative ion air purifier should achieve the following:

- Remove pollutants from the air: Ionic air purifiers (ionizers) contain negative ion generators that charge airborne particles so they become attracted to and settle on room surfaces or purifier plates, effectively removing harmful particles from the air you breathe. In the March 2000 issue of *Agricultural Research Magazine,* researchers at the U.S. Department of Agriculture reported that ionic air purifiers reduced salmonella (bacteria) transmission in a poultry housed (where extremely high levels of air pollution are normally found) between chicks by 98%; airborne salmonella (bacteria) by 95% and airborne dust and particles by 99% in 60 seconds.

- Negatively charged air: In 1974, the Swiss Meteorological Institute first studied problems related to seasonal winds in various regions of the earth. The Foehn that blows across Switzerland, the Sirocco in Italy, the Sharav in the Middle East, and the Mistral in southern France were found to cause physical and mental effects ranging from headaches and depression to heart attacks.

The one common denominator in all of these wind variants was the type of electrical charge of the ions in the air. A very high concentration of positive ions was found to be the culprit. Conversely, the air quality studied at the site of a waterfall, in the mountains, at beaches or after a spring rain showed significant amounts of negative ions. Further research revealed that human beings respond to negative ion levels above 1000 ions per cc.

Scientific research concluded that negatively charged ions have positive effects on living organisms. Plants grow faster and healthier, lab animals are calmed and more able to perform certain tasks and humans respond with increased alertness and relaxation.

French physicist J. Bricard discovered the relationship between the electrical charge of the air and its micro pollution as early as the 1950s. The physical law of Bricard is simple: Low concentration of negative ions in the air equals pollution. High concentration of negative ions equals healthy air.

- Increased oxygen intake: Research about negative ions has been conducted since the 1950s and studies have shown that exposure to negative ions results in improvement in mood, anxiety, cognitive ability, energy, depression and sleep quality, as well as improvement in breathing and air quality. With increased oxygen intake from negative ions, one gets a feeling of alertness and vitality, similar to the feeling we get when we are in a beautiful forest or near a thundering waterfall or breathing crisp, clean mountain air.

In PingLongevity™, unless you're living in a place with superior air quality, we recommend installing negative ion air purifiers in all rooms where you spend a great deal time, including your living space, office and automobile if you happen to drive a lot on polluted city streets.

2.8   DIETARY SUPPLEMENTATION

We believe dietary supplements are necessary, primarily because our fruits, vegetables and grains are grown in soils that have been overused and are nutrient depleted. Livestock is fed artificial food. According to the latest U.S. Department of Agriculture food tables, there has been a huge decrease in the nutritional value of food over the last 40 years.

Taking spinach as an example, in the past four decades, its content of vitamin C has been reduced by 45%, vitamin A by 17.1%, calcium by 6.5%, potassium by 18.7% and magnesium by 10.2%.

Because of the depletion of nutrients in our food, it is important to supplement our diets with essential nutrients.

However, we are all faced with difficult decisions and confusing expert advice and marketing pitches:

- Which brand should we choose? In the book *Comparative Guide to Nutritional Supplements* by Lyle MacWilliam, hundreds of multi-vitamins and minerals were compared. The top 10 brands were chosen as: Essentials, Ultra Preventive X, Extend Plus, Life Force Multiple, Basic Mindell Plus, Life Extension Mix, Maxxum 4, Super Complete, Ultra Preventive Beta, Multiguard, Forward Multi-Nutrient. If you check other books, you may encounter a completely different list of recommendations. So it's confusing, right?

- Which supplements do you take? You're told many things are good for you: multi-vitamins and minerals, fish oil, calcium, garlic, carnitine, CoQ10, taurine, CLA, chromium, DHEA, tyrosine, biotin, magnesium, resveratrol, black cohosh, pygeum, glutamine, cinnamon, niacin, zinc, green tea, fiber, iodoral, DIM, saw palmetto, isoflavones, chrysin, muira rama, nettle, lipoic acid, silymarin and lecithin, just to name a few. Everything is good for you. Pretty soon, you are up to 50–100 pills each day.

Are there any side effects from taking supplements? What exactly do you need? What's the correct philosophy and approach to supplementation?

2.8.1   Nutritional Medicine and Risks from the Dietary Supplement Industry

Modern manufacturing technologies are now able to single out an ingredient from a natural food or plant and extract it into a highly concentrated product, usually hundreds of times more potent than natural whole foods. Care must be taken when using these highly concentrated dietary supplements.

For example, tofu or other whole soybean products, as whole

foods, are a 5,000-year-old tradition in Asia and proven to be healthy and safe. Soy is not only a complete protein source, but it also contains phytoestrogens called isoflavones, which together with the whole food have substantial health benefits.

The dietary supplement industry has rolled out many concentrated isoflavone products. Usually on a dry weight basis, raw soybeans contain between 2 and 4 milligrams of total isoflavones per gram. Soy-based foods differ somewhat in their concentration of isoflavones, but all of the traditional soy foods, such as tofu, soymilk, tempeh and miso are rich sources of isoflavones providing about 30 to 40 milligrams per serving. Typical dietary soy and isoflavone extracts, for example, Ultra Soy Extract of Life Extension, contain as high as 1250 mg isoflavones per serving! This is about 40 times the potency of the natural food! Many of you, even some in medical professions think natural supplements are safe. However, with such potency, they can have a significant impact on the body. Like drugs, used correctly, supplements can have a positive effect, but the opposite can be true, too.

Phytoestrogens have a weak estrogenic effect. When you take them in whole foods, they are safe and healthy. But when you take them in highly concentrated amounts in supplements, care must be taken because they may change your hormone balance—to the good or bad!

Similarly, flaxseed as a whole food is a wonder food, full of health benefits. But now you may choose to take supplements rather than the whole flaxseeds. Just 1 gram (2 capsules) of supplements can be equivalent to as many as 70 grams of whole flaxseeds in lignan contents. Lignan is the major phytoestrogen in flaxseeds! Again, there will be measurable impact on hormone balance—good or bad. Care must be taken to make sure you are on the good side.

Another example: Leading authorities are advocating red yeast rice as an effective way to lower cholesterol as an alternative to the statin drugs. There are many red yeast rice-based dietary supplements on the market. However, do you know that the primary ingredient in these red yeast rice supplements, lovastatin, is also the exact active pharmaceutical ingredient in prescription statin drugs for high cholesterol such as Mevacor, Lipitor, Zocor, Levacor and Pravachol? In fact, lovastatin was originally derived from a type of red yeast called Monascus rubber. For these prescription drugs, there have been many known side effects, including liver damage with long-term use. Taking a large dose of red yeast rice supplements can have side effects similar to prescription drugs, since the concentration in modern supplements has become so high. Indeed, "natural" does not mean "safe."

A new study conducted by researchers of University of Auckland and published in the *British Medical Journal* found that calcium supplementation increases the risk of heart attack.

> "Previous research suggested they (calcium supplements) might also protect against vascular disease by cutting blood cholesterol levels.
>
>   After a careful analysis of the data, the researchers confirmed 36 heart attacks in 31 women who took the supplements, compared with 22 heart attacks in 21 women who took the placebo.
>
>   The researchers said the supplements may raise the risk of a heart attack by accelerating hardening of the blood vessels."
> —*BBC NEWS*, JAN. 16, 2008

You may notice that studies with contradictory conclusions are often reported. For example, scientists studying calcium supplementation should be exploring the question of why calcium is absorbed by the bones or why it is not. If calcium is not absorbed, the arteries can get calcified. There are several explanations why someone is not absorbing calcium, even though there is sufficient calcium intake. There could be a lack of vitamin D, a hormone imbalance in the testosterone-estrogen axis or a decline of parathyroid hormones.

Yes, modern technologies can do wonders. But if you're not careful, and think that you can just take supplements and get the same nutrition as in really good whole foods, you may be wrong!

In general, except for a class we call functional foods, we should treat most modern dietary supplements, including concentrated herbal medicines, as drugs. When taking them, you must know what you're doing. This is why a new discipline of medicine has emerged. Doctors use highly concentrated nutritional supplements to treat very serious diseases. These supplements, used properly, can be very effective, and can have fewer side effects than synthetic drugs.

2.8.2   The Functional Food Approach to Supplementation

The PingLongevity™ Diet looks at dietary supplements with two purposes. We use them for disease treatment and sub-health reversal. We also use them for basic food supplementation.

There is a class of supplements we call functional foods. These are concentrates of the nutrients of entire *whole foods* such as vegetables and fruits, while the bulky starch and sugar have been removed. These are the ones we use for regular supplementation. The renowned nutritional scientist Colin Campbell said in his best selling book, *The China Study*, "Nutrition represents the combined activities of countless food substances. The whole is greater than the sum of its parts." Nature knows how to combine thousands of nutrients. When a single element of a nutrient is separated out by humans, it is difficult to balance and to achieve the integrated effect."

Therefore, the approach of supplementation in the Ping-Longevity™ Diet is to use only low temperature produced, high quality organic whole functional food supplements. Care must be taken to select only the best quality brands. Functional foods must be processed at very low temperatures to preserve the food enzymes as discussed in Section 2.1.

The food supplements that everyone needs are:

- A vegetable extract: A good product can pack over 200 lbs of whole green essence into a bottle of highly concentrated vegetable nutrients at less than 12 calories per serving. Research indicates that regular supplementation with these products can reduce biological age for the 28–40 age group by 6 years and for the 41–65 age group by 13.5 years.

- A high ORAC value fruit extract: The new scientific breakthrough in nutritional circles is ORAC™ (Oxygen Radical Absorbance Capacity), an index developed to measure the antioxidant power of nutrients. A good fruit supplement must be a special blend that contains at the very least the wonder fruits like blueberry, cranberry, apple, raspberry, concord grape, strawberry, watermelon, bilberry, blood orange, apple pectin, white cherry extract, pomegranate extract, blueberry extract, prune extract, red wine extract, resveratrol, vitamin C, beta carotene, green tea and grape seed extracts. Each serving contains no less than 5000 ORAC. It must be manufactured with a low temp process to preserve all the nutrients and enzymes.

- A protein extract: A good protein could be both vegetable based and whey based. It must be produced at a low temperature to preserve all the enzymes and nutrients. For example, the following nutrients in natural proteins are usually lacking in protein supplements because of high temp processes: beta-lactoglobulin, alpha-lactalbumin, immunoglobulins, glycomacropeptide, bovine serum albumin, lactogerrin, lactoperoxidase, lysozyme, and many growth factors.

- Fish oil has multiple benefits and should be an essential supplement. However, quality varies very much in the market. Be careful to choose pharmaceutical grade fish oil, each softgel containing at least 400 mg of EPA, 200 mg of DHA, sourced from Norway—the cleanest water, processed only without organs, molecularly distilled to eliminate all environmental contaminants and manufactured by a reputable maker.

- A high potency multi-antioxidant: Research has shown that many antioxidants are more effective and better able to ward off cellular damage when present in balanced combinations. There are reasons why you need a balanced mix. A good multi-antioxidant should contain: resveratrol, proanthocyanadins (OPC), polyphenols, carotenoids, curcuminoids, bioflavonoids and terpenes, chlorophyll, phytosterols, isothiocyanates and sulforaphanes, alpha lipoic acid and n-acetylcysteine.

- Eat super foods: We also supplement our meals with whole high nutritional density foods such as raw cold milled flaxseed, wheat germ, chia seeds, quinoa and high nutrition herbs such as goji berry, polygonum and American ginseng.

2.8.3   The MVA Test

"Essential vitamins and minerals, as well as amino acids are like the alphabet. If you miss several letters, you will lose a lot of words—some important building blocks of the body!"

—Dr. Ping Wu

"For many years, I have had large intestine ulcers and other gastrointestinal symptoms. I've seen many doctors who can offer no cures. Doctors told me I have autoimmune disease, leaky gut syndrome and many other possible illnesses. Basically, there's no treatment that works. Finally, I went to Dr. Ping. In the checkup, she found that I'm low in many essential amino acids. My dark field live blood showed money-string like blood cells all sticking together and dry blood showed lots of white spaces. However, I do not have protease deficiency. Apparently a lack of many essential proteins makes me unable to provide building blocks for many body repair mechanisms. Somehow I could not absorb proteins, no matter how much I ate. Dr. Ping put me on a very high quality, super fine absorbable whey protein supplement. Within a matter of a few weeks, my symptoms start to get better. Upon a follow-up endoscopic examination, my ulcers had nearly healed."

—Jennifer, Los Angeles

The MVA test measures mineral, vitamin and amino acid levels. Even with a good diet and food supplementation, for various reasons, we may still be unable to absorb the nutrients, so we become deficient in certain essential elements. This may have severe negative impact on our bodies, since "essential" means our bodies cannot make these substances and we must get them from foods so they can be absorbed and digested.

2.9   FOOD ANTIBODIES AND ALLERGIES

Most of us think of food allergies as the severe ones where people are rushed to emergency rooms for life threatening conditions. There's another type of food allergy, a silent type that is so prevalent that almost all of us have it. This kind of food intolerance does not result in a severe reaction. These intolerances build up over time. Many times they are the result of years of overeating one type of food. The body is overloaded on the food and the immune system starts to attack itself each time such food is taken. When the immune system is busy dealing with these essentially harmless foods, the total body immune capability to deal with real external threats becomes compromised, leading to many symptoms and syndromes seemingly unrelated to food allergy.

Type one, or "classic," allergies cause redness, swelling, bloating, diarrhea, constipation and heat in the body as a result of the elevated blood levels of immunoglobulin E (IgE). Less than 5% of the population has severe acute type one allergic reactions. However, contrary to popular belief, the symptoms produced by IgE can be subtle and similar to those seen in delayed allergy reactions.

The other type of food allergy is a delayed reaction one with an antibody called immunoglobulin G (IgG). This type of food intolerance or sensitivity has a delayed onset and is typically less acute, but occurs considerably more often. Symptoms can seem to be quite unrelated to the foods, for example, irritable bowel, autism, cystic fibrosis, rheumatoid arthritis, epilepsy, sleeplessness after eating, skin rash, joint ache, weight gain, diabetes, asthma and sinusitis.

"My son Brian is a 21-year-old Berkley student. In the past few months, Brian's immune system has dramatically declined. He was one of the rare patients who had the H1N1 flu virus twice. The constant viral infection and bacterial attack has caused so much down time that Brian had to be on leave from college. He consulted many specialists, but nothing helped. His tests showed nothing significant except for low immunoglobulin. They put him on antibiotics whenever there's an infection. He's been on the drug every month! The poor kid was so weak, low energy and depressed that he talked hopelessly about dropping out of school.

I've been a patient of Dr. Ping for many years, so I took Brian to her office. Dr. Ping performed a thorough diagnosis and prescribed several medical tests. When the results came back, one of the tests, IgE and IgG food antigen test, showed Brian to be severely allergic to eggs and dairy products.

'Are you allergic to eggs and milk?' asked Dr. Ping.

'Not at all. They're a part of my daily diet,' replied Brian.

Apparently there were few discernable symptoms when Brian ate eggs and dairy products. But when Brian stopped eating eggs and dairy, it took just a couple of weeks for his symptoms to disappear and for him to be back in school.

Three months later, Brian went to see Dr. Ping. He looked wonderful, had lost 25 pounds and he was back to working out at the gym every day."

—JAMES, BRIAN'S FATHER, ORANGE COUNTY, CA

"For over 10 years, I have chronic sinus problem. Every few weeks, I'd get sinus congestion and infection, which causes a severe headache. I've been to many specialists. A dentist took out my wisdom teeth on both sides. A nose, ear, throat doctor took out my tonsils. I also tried TCM, using certain herbs for treatment. Despite all of this, my problem continued. Finally, I met with a famous doctor who specializes in sinus related diseases. He sent me for a CT scan and decided I was borderline for surgery because there is narrowing in certain places and those narrow spots are easily clogged and the clogged areas become a haven for infection-causing bacteria. But his diagnosis was that it was not yet severe enough to warrant surgery.

'Sorry, there's really no cure,' the doctor told me. 'You'll have to live with this for the rest of your life and use antibiotics every time you get an infection.' He'd then prescribe a two-week course of high potency antibiotics for me. He explained that the sinuses are difficult to treat with antibiotics, so it would be necessary to use stronger ones for a longer time each time I got an infection. Well, with the frequency of infections I had, I would need to use antibiotics every other month! How can this be a solution?

A friend asked me to try Dr. Ping. With her thorough diagnosis, Dr. Ping was pretty sure that despite my narrower sinus cavities, my problem was most likely due to delayed food allergy, so I went through IgG testing. The result was a long list of foods to which I'm allergic, including tofu, eggs, milk, red pepper, lobster, walnut, beans and corn. These are my favorite foods!

'How can I live without these foods?' I asked Dr. Ping.

'You may have been eating these foods for a lot of years. Over time, your body gradually developed antibodies to them. The reaction builds up and manifests itself in your weakest spot, i.e., your sinus. You may want to stop eating these foods for a while or at least with much less frequency. Later, once you're better, you may be able to get back to some of the foods,' Dr. Ping suggested.

I stopped eating the list of foods. Since then, for the last two years, I've seldom been sick. My sinus problem magically went away! Ten years of sinus pain is cured!"

—ERIC, ORANGE COUNTY, CA

"A 60-year-old school teacher, J., has been suffering from chronic fatigue, low thyroid function, bloating and hypoglycemia after eating. She is overweight and had been unable to lose weight. She could not follow a diet because when she did not eat, she felt dizzy due to low blood sugar. After she stopping eating a few foods that tested positive in her IgG and IgE, she has seen her blood sugar stabilize and does not experience food cravings anymore. Without dieting and supplements, she lost 35 pounds effortlessly. Her other symptoms largely went away as well."

—DR. PING

In industrialized nations, farmed and genetically engineered food, processed food and environmental waste seem to have caused a dramatic increase in food intolerance. For example, additives used in prepared foods have been found to be particularly problematic. Results of a multi-disciplinary study of autistic kids showed that all of the subjects had at least some reactivity to food colorings. Similarly, many chemical containing foods are intolerogenic. Salicylates, for example, occur in many fruits and vegetables and can induce a pharmacologically mediated adverse reaction. Dietary lectins, which may be resistant to degradation through cooking and digestion, occur in numerous vegetables, fruits, grains and some meats. A "leaky gut" whose failure to degrade food components, may occur when undigested proteins traverse the gut prematurely and enter the circulation. It is sometimes seen that reactions to apples do not occur unless there are simultaneous high levels of airborne birch pollen, which cross reacts with apple.

A food that contains an intolerogenic chemical may be tolerated in moderation, but become intolerable by immune systems when consumed on a more frequent basis.

In a good diet plan, such as the PingLongevity™ Diet, it is very important to exclude all the foods that test IgE and IgG positive. Most of the time, these are foods that you've been overeating for many years. Your system may have been fatigued by the challenge of these foods, resulting in a compromised immune system. Reducing or eliminating these foods may resolve many sub-health problems, even some severe degenerative illness.

2.10 DETOXIFICATION

We are being bombarded with toxins on a continuous basis. Although our bodies have their built in detoxification mechanisms, in the liver and kidneys, our systems may not be able to handle the overload from our modern industrialized environment. Frequent use of detoxification protocols may help prevent this overload.

2.10.1 Sources of Toxins

Prescription drugs bring a significant toxin load into the body. Most drugs function via only one specific mechanism. By affecting just one metabolic pathway, imbalances can develop in the body that often result in dangerous side effects.

For example, anti-inflammatory drugs that inhibit the cyclooxygenase-2 (COX-2) enzyme have shown the ability to relieve arthritis. However, a study published in the August 2000 issue of the *Journal of Immunology* identifies a potential long-term problem with this enzyme that could lead to cartilage and tissue degeneration. Another example is that synthetic estrogen used in hormone replacement therapy may lead to endometrial cancer in women. Antibiotics are shown to harm the tendons. Millions of people have tried the diabetes wonder drug, Rezulin, the silicone breast implant and statin drugs, to name just a few, only to find significant and sometimes fatal side effects.

In general, drug toxicity affects the liver and kidneys most often. When the liver malfunctions, hormone balance is also impaired because many hormones, such as estrogen, are processed through the liver.

"I used it because I have to, not because I like the side effects," most people would say. Indeed, life is full of compromise, isn't it? On the other hand, what if we don't "have to"? In the 5,000 year-old Chinese medicine tradition, it was said that top medicine optimizes people who are healthy, middle medicine heals people who are in sub-health and low medicine treats people who are sick.

In PingLongevity™, we first ask you to live the most health-optimizing lifestyle possible. Then we use herbal medicine, nutritional medicine, detoxification and hormone balance to treat your sub-health and illness. Drugs, due to their toxicity, are always the last resort.

"Patients, husband and wife, both had high blood glucose levels and regularly took diabetes drugs. I told them about the side effects and explained the benefits of a healthy diet, but they answered, 'We're in our 70s, why should we suffer by not eating what we like?'

Well, last fall, they came to visit us and stayed in town for a couple of months. Simply by eating a healthier diet with us, now both of them are off the drugs.

'We learned how you guys eat. Now we don't even want to go back to our previous diet. It feels so good!' said my patients.

Type 2 diabetes drugs for controlling blood sugar level have severe side effects, such as raising heart attack risks by as much as 40%, lung fluid build-up, hypoglycemia and potential drug toxicity overloading the liver and body's detoxification pathways."

—DR. PING WU

Environmental toxins are another serious problem:

"Environmental pollution is major category of toxins. Bad air: We speculated that nanoparticles in automobile exhaust have a causal relationship with brain tumors. In the lab, we then found that even the brain cells of laboratory mice undergo a transition to suggest preconditions to converting to cancer when subjected to the type of air found on and around freeways, after just a few short months of exposure."

—DR. KEITH BLACK

Man-made electromagnetic waves are environmental toxins of increasing danger levels. There are many controversial studies about cell phones. Some believe the RF waves through the antenna on your cell phone can cause brain tumors. Others think its risk is minimal. You may have noticed that if you drive your car with the radio on and you drive under or near a high voltage transmission line, your radio reception is disrupted. What if some of us live or work very close to such transmission lines?

Food is another source of chemicals and toxins. For example, nitrates are used as preservatives to help prevent the growth of bacteria that cause botulism and other food borne illnesses. These nitrates would break down, forming nitrites. Eventually, nitrites themselves were added directly to the meat to speed up the curing process. Nitrites continue to be used in cooked meats, such as preserved meats, hot dogs, bacon and cured ham to maintain the traditional pink color and cured flavor. Nitrites contribute to the formation of potentially dangerous carcinogens in the body, which can result in malignant tumor growth.

Pesticides and other chemicals in fruits and vegetables, antibiotics and hormones in livestock are all toxins we're exposed to on a daily basis.

Heavy metal is another toxin to which you can be exposed through your food, with many detrimental effects on our body. Due to industrial pollution of coastlines, seafood can be a major source of heavy metal, especially large fish at the top of the food chain, as seen in the table below.

MERCURY IN SEAFOOD	
MERCURY IN FISH TISSUE (AVERAGE PARTS PER MILLION)	**SPECIES**
0.97–1.9	Tile fish
0.48–0.97	Sword fish, king mackerel, shark, orange roughy, salt water bass, moonfish
0.32–0.48	Marlin, trout
0.24–0.32	Tuna, lobster, grouper, bluefish
0.12–0.24	Canned tuna, halibut, pollock, Dungeness crab, mahi mahi, Atlantic cod, haddock, whitefish, herring
0.08–0.12	King crab, perch
Under 0.8	Salmon, shrimp, clam, oyster, tilapia, scallop, catfish, flounder, sole

Source: U.S. Environmental Protection Agency (EPA), U.S. Food and Drug Administration (FDA)

Heavy metal can also come from many other industrial products to which we are exposed every day, as seen in the table on page 96.

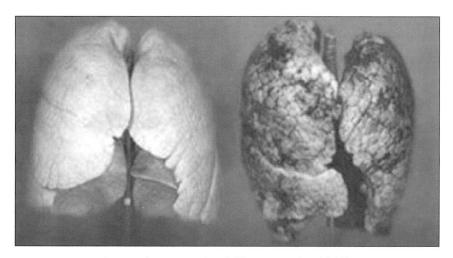

Lungs of a non-smoker (left) vs. a smoker (right)

We all know that cigarettes are highly toxic to the lungs. There's enough information about the effect. Without the need for further elaboration, you only need to look the lungs of a non-smoker compared to a smoker to understand the harmful effects of smoking (see the picture above).

Alcohol is also toxic to the liver. Alcoholic liver disease is one of the most serious medical consequences of chronic alcohol use. Moreover, chronic excessive alcohol use is the single most important cause of illness and death from liver disease (alcoholic hepatitis and cirrhosis) in the United States. Alcohol also has a very negative effect on hormones. For example, studies of alcohol's effects on male reproduction have been conducted in rats because the rat model mimics the human male reproductive system. Research has demonstrated that both acute and chronic alcohol exposure are associated with low levels of hypothalamic LHRH and pituitary LH in the adult and pubertal male rat and further studies have suggested that alcohol inhibits testosterone secretion by the testes as well.

There are many more sources of toxins. For example, simply by overeating, you create undigested foods and wastes, which put burden on the body as toxins.

HEAVY METAL FROM OTHER SOURCES

ALUMINUM

Alum
Aluminum cans
Aluminum cookware
Aluminum dust
Aluminum foil
Aluminum phosphate
Aluminum silicate
Animal feed
Antacids
Automotive parts
Automotive exhaust
Baking powder
Beer
American cheese
Ceramics
Cigarettes filters
Cool combustion
Color additives
Construction materials
Dental amalgams
Deodorants
Drinking water
Insulated wiring
Nasal spray
Medical compounds
Milk products
Pesticides
Table salt
Tobacco smoke
Toothpaste
Vanilla powder

ARSENIC

Animal feed
Automobile exhaust
Cool combusting
Colored chalk
Herbicides
Household detergents
Industrial dust
Insecticides
Seafood
Wallpaper
Water, city and well
Wine
Wood preservatives

CADMIUM

Alloys, dental
Batteries
Tools
Marine hardware
Cadmium vapor lamps
Candy
Ceramics
Cereals, refined
Cigarette smoke
Cisterns
Colas
Copper refineries
Electroplating
Fertilizers, phosphate
Fungicides

Grains, refined
Incineration of tires,
   rubber, plastics
Iron roofs
Kidney
Liver
Marijuana
Milk, evaporated
Oil, motor
Oysters
Point pigments
Pesticides
Pipes, galvanized
Plastics, polyvinyl
Processed foods
Silver polish
Electric blankets
Soft drinks
Solders
Vending machine
Water, city
Welding metal
Water, softened
Water, well

LEAD

Bone meal
Canned fruit/juice
Care batteries
Cigarette ash
Cool combustion

Eating utensils

Exhaust, auto

Hair dyes

Lead pipes

Lead refineries

Lead smelters

Liver

Mascara

Milk, also evaporated

Newsprint

Organ meats

Paint

Pesticides

Produce near roads

Putty

PVC containers

Rainwater

Snow

Tobacco

Toothpaste

Toys

Water, city

Water, well

Wine

NICKEL

Coal combustion

Exhaust, auto

Fertilizers

Super phosphate

Food processing

Hydrogenated fats, oils

Industrial waste

Stainless steel cookware

Baking powder

MERCURY

Adhesives

Air conditioner filters

Body powders, talc

Broken thermometers

Cosmetics

Dental fillings

Diuretics

Fabric softeners

Felt

Floor waxes/polishes

Fungicides

Industrial waste

Laxatives

Mercurochrome

Points

Photoengraving

Psoriatic ointments

Seafood

Sewage disposal

Skin lightening cream

Suppositories

Tanning leather

Tattooing

Wood preservatives

RADIATION

X-Rays

Computers

Microwave

Nuclear testing

Electric high power lines

Rubber carpet backing

Cancer treatments

Food irradiation

Electro-magnetic radiation

Atmospheric radiation from a weakened ionosphere

COPPER

Beer

Copper cookware

Chocolate

Copper IUD's

Rate poisons

Copper pipes

Dental, prosthesis

Fungicides

Hemodialysis

Ice makers

Industrial wastes

Insecticides

Liver

Milk

Nuts

Oysters

Source: *Surviving a Toxic Crisis,* by William Kellas, Ph.D.

2.10.2 Detoxification

There are medical grade detoxification programs, but like in nutritional medicine, you need to consult with a trained professional. For self-managed cleansing programs, you may consider the following:

- The body's own cleaning mechanism: If you allow yourself 2 to 4 hours each day with completely empty stomach and intestines, i.e., feeling hungry, your body will sweep itself clean.

- Avoid foods with chemicals:
  - Use ionic air purifiers in bedroom, office and cars where you spend most of your time;
  - Use high quality ionic water purifier;
  - Use a high quality ozone cleaner to clean fruits and vegetables prior to eating. Alternatively, use 1 part of white vinegar, 3 parts of water for cleaning;
  - Avoid eating large ocean fish such as tilefish, swordfish, shark, king mackerel, orange roughy, sea bass, moonfish, marlin and tuna.
  - Avoid farmed fish;
  - Eat organic foods;
  - Avoid processed foods;

- Avoid chemical products: Use natural products in place of chemicals for household cleaning, including detergents, degreasers, lawn and garden chemicals.

- Use corded earphones when talking on the cell phone for more than 15 minutes;

- Avoid prolonged exposure to high voltage electrical transmission lines;

- Periodically perform liver, intestine, blood and lymph detoxification. Doctors usually use high bio-available natural dietary supplements and certain equipments such as far infrared saunas.

2.11 SUMMARY

In this Chapter, we discussed the main principles of the Ping-Longevity™ Diet:

- Diet: The healthiest longevity foods have the following characteristics: *live, fresh and raw, high nutritional density, low glycemic index, alkaline forming.*

- Eat only when you're hungry. Be aware of food order. Take fruits first, soup second, other main course last.

- Air and water: We recommend using ionic air filters and ionic alkaline purified water.

- Food Antigens: To avoid provoking an immune response from foods, test for food allergies, especially IgG, the silent, chronic food allergy. Rotate foods in your diet to prevent building food intolerances.

- Supplementation: Use functional food supplements, vegetables, fruits, proteins, fish oils and high nutritional density foods such as raw milled flaxseeds. Unless prescribed by a nutritional medicine doctor, avoid using too many dietary supplements.

- Detoxification: Detox every day to prevent toxins from building up.

- Undergo MVA testing to make sure you're not lacking any essential minerals, vitamins and amino acids.

The more you can incorporate these foods into your diet, the longer, healthier and happier your life will be. You will lose unwanted weight, gain considerable energy and get back your youthful body shape.

The list found on page 100 offers some examples of good food choices.

Using these foods, you may come up with your own customized recipes. See page 102 for an example of healthy recipes.

PINGLONGEVITY™ FOODS (RANKED IN ORDER OF PREFERENCE)

VEGETABLES (raw and organic)

Sea vegetables
Asparagus
Broccoli
Beets
Cauliflower
Bell peppers
Kale
Swiss chard
Turnip greens
Carrots
Celery
Tomatoes
Eggplant
Collard greens
Cabbage
Cucumbers
Fennel
Leeks
Mushrooms, crimini
Mushrooms, shiitake
Mustard greens
Onions
Parsley
Romaine lettuce
Spinach
Squash, summer
Squash, winter

FRUITS (organic)

Blueberries
Apples
Kiwifruit
Noni
Plums
Cranberries
Pears
Raspberries
Strawberries
Watermelon

SPICES AND DRESSINGS

Lemon/limes
Apple vinegar (raw)
Ginger (raw)
Garlic
Chili Pepper, dried
Honey (raw)
Soy sauce (tamari)
Sea salt (raw)
Olive oil, extra virgin
Olives in oil
Papaya (raw)
Pineapple (raw)
Omega-3 fish oil (raw)

FOOD FOR ENERGY (replacing grains)

Avocadoes
Chia Seeds
Flax seeds (raw)
Wheat germ (raw)
Wheat grass
Quinoa seeds (raw/cooked)
Corn (raw & young)
Bean sprouts (raw)
Yams (raw or baked)
Sweet potatoes (raw or baked)
Potatoes (raw)
Miso
Tofu
Pumpkin seeds
Sesame seeds
Walnuts
Sunflower seeds
Almonds
Peanuts

SUPPLEMENTS (high quality)

Mixed greens
High ORAC mixed fruits
Fish oil
Proteins
High potency antioxidant mix
Digestive enzymes (pre-meal)

FISH* (raw, deep-sea)

*Avoid large fish
Salmon
Flounder
Sole
Salmon eggs
Shrimp
Scallop
Oyster
Nishimoto Salted Jelly Fish

DAIRY (organic)

Milk, goat (fat-free & raw)
Milk (fat-free & raw)
Yogurt (fat-free & unpasteurized)
Eggs (raw or medium rare)
Cheese (fat-free & unpasteurized)

HERBS

Wolfberry (raw)
American ginseng (raw)
He Shou Wu (raw)

WATER

Alkaline water
Green tea
Spring water

You may wonder if you can follow the kind of diet described here. The idea is to take one step at a time. Try to be creative. If you are not able to eat all of these foods raw, start by using the raw ingredients to make healthy sauces and seasonings. You don't have to use any specific recipes. Make dishes that suit your own taste.

To begin the transition to better foods, you can also avoid eating refined foods and those with a high glycemic index. At times, you may still want to eat "junk" food. Do so to satisfy your body (or really your mind!), but always take pre-meal enzymes, use insulin-sensitivity-reducing herbs (to reduce the meal's glycemic index) and skip or lighten the next meals so that your system can clean itself out completely right away.

Make sure that when you eat, your stomach is completely empty (you will feel hungry). Gradually, you will find yourself adapting to cleaner, more energetic food over just a few months. You will crave less and less of the foods in the "less desirable" category. Let the transition take place naturally.

PINGLONGEVITY™ SAMPLE RECIPES

RECIPES FOR YOUR HEALTHY DAYS (AT LEAST 5 DAYS PER WEEK)

MEAL	FOODS	PINGLONGEVITY™ FOODS
Daily Detox	Alkaline water	Alkaline water
Breakfast	PingLongevity™ Foods Mix	Soy milk or fat-free raw milk, flax seeds, wheat germ, chia seeds, wolfberry, he shou wu,
	Supplements	green mix, fruit mix, protein
Lunch	Yam/sweet potato	Yam or sweet potato
	Corn	Corns
	Vegetable drink	Vegetables in PingLongevity™ Foods
	Eggs	Organic eggs
	Nuts	Nuts in PingLongevity™ Foods
Snacks	Afternoon fruits	Choose among fruits in PingLongevity™ Foods
	Energy foods	avocado, papaya, mango
Dinner	Vegetable salad	Choose among vegetables in PingLongevity™ Foods
	Broccoli salad	Broccoli or cauliflower
	Sashimi salad	Seafood in PingLongevity™ Foods
	Salmon egg salad	Raw sushi-grade salmon eggs
	Steamed fish	Fresh rock or sole fish

RECIPES FOR YOUR FREE DAYS (AT MOST 2 DAYS PER WEEK)

Free-day meal		Any of your favorite restaurants or home cooked meals

RECIPE

1–3 glasses at least 1 hour before meal, or at least 2 hours after meal

Mix with a food mixer

Use high-quality ones with food

Baked

Raw, young/juicy

Raw blended, adjust taste: papaya & carrots for sweet, lime for sour, etc.

Boiled (medium/rare)

Baked or soaked (for 24 hours)

Eat raw

Eat raw

Dressing: lime or apple vinegar for sour, papaya or pineapple or raw honey for sweet, dried raw hot chili pepper for spiciness, fish oil for extra taste & nutrition

Raw; sauce preparation: Tamari soy sauce, garlic, green onions, chili pepper, honey

Thinly sliced fish, use on top or mix with vegetable salad

Use on top or mix with vegetable salad

Mix water, soy sauce, honey, ginger, green onions, garlic, sea salt. Steam in a sauce pan, fish fillet on top, for 10 mins.

Take digestive enzymes before the meal. Skip 1–2 meals before or after eating a large "free-day" meal. Gradually reduce processed, refined, overcooked, fried, sweet, salty foods and soft drinks, alcohol, cigarettes, farmed animal foods, non-organic foods, satuated and trans fats.

CHAPTER 3

Maximize Metabolic Efficiency

In this chapter, we'll discuss caloric restriction as the only scientif-ically proven way of extending your lifespan. To start with let's perform a simple experiment and think about its deep implications in regards to youthfulness and longevity:

The Rose Experiment

You may have noticed that florists like to keep roses and other flow-ers in refrigerators. Why? Of course, so they will last longer.

Go to buy two sets of identical roses. When you get home, put set #1 in your own refrigerator, which has a similar temperature setting as the florist's and set #2 in your living room at room temperature. Furthermore, add some plant food to the vase for set #2. Then observe which set blooms first, and which one dies out first. The result is, of course, set #2.

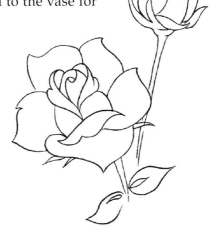

What does this tell us? Apparently, the life of a rose has something to do with how fast it lives its own life. For roses, temperature and additional plant food can accelerate the aging process. In humans, the rate at which we burn calories affects the speed of aging. In this chapter, we'll discuss the only scientifically proven way to extend maximum lifespan, namely, caloric restriction. We'll tell you how Ping-Longevity™ Caloric Restriction will help you extend your young and productive lifespan.

3.1   METABOLIC RATE—THE RATE OF LIVING

In this chapter, we will show you how to lower your metabolic rate to achieve a more efficient body. One very effective way of lowering metabolic rate is through caloric restriction, so that will be the focus of our discussion.

You may immediately wonder why we want you to lower your metabolic rate. Isn't that true that you have been told by many experts to increase your metabolic rate through growth hormones replacement and other methods? Even herbalists talk about how the Chinese herbs accelerate metabolic rate.

Much expert advice centers around increasing your metabolic rate to be more "healthy." Titles like "10 Ways to Boost Your Metabolism" are everywhere on the airwaves and in the press. They say that if caloric intake is dropped consistently below a certain level, the body will enter a state of starvation. Therefore, it would slow down its basal metabolic rate. Hence, it'll lose less weight. These experts advise instead, we should focus on increasing our metabolism rather than on reducing caloric intake.

As you read through this chapter, you'll understand that the advice to increase your metabolic rate, unless you have hypothyroidism, is wrong. Instead, you should lower your metabolic rate by making your body a more efficient engine. This is apparent if you think about the Rose Experiment above.

Now, to aid your understanding, let's do another experiment:

The Car Experiment

Suppose someone has convinced you that you should at least burn five gallons of gasoline a day with your brand new BMW. However, your average use of a car to go to work, shopping, gym, etc. is about three gallons a day. In order to burn five gallons a day, you have to "work" the car each night, by driving it aimlessly around the town. After about a week, you may wonder why you're doing this. Is it a good thing? After all, your car will wear out faster. The engine will pile up higher mileage and the car will have a lower resale value.

Is this a dumb story? Then think about how many people needlessly burn calories through exercise every day.

Metabolism represents all of the body's chemical processes, growth, repair and digestion. It is divided into anabolic (the growth and repair) process and catabolic (decomposition) process and is indirectly related to heart rate, body temperature and caloric intake. Metabolic rate is defined as calories burned per gram of body mass per day.

Metabolic rate is the rate of living: how fast you live through your limited life potential. The speed at which you can walk 100 miles depends on your pace. Conceptually, if you live at a faster rate, you end your life sooner, given that you only have a finite capacity to live, according to the law of life.

A car may run 150,000 miles before the engine dies. You can maintain your car by changing the oil, tuning up the engine and replacing the brakes, but it still has a finite number of miles to run. If you burn gas to increase your speed, the car will break down sooner. Why? The reason is that burning gas or cleaning the engine is never 100% effective. There are always deposits, oxidization and rust plus mechanical wear and tear.

Similarly, people burn fuel with the aid of the oxygen they breathe. The process is not 100% efficient. The byproduct when burning fuel (glucose) with the aid of oxygen gradually kills the living body systems through oxidation as the repair mechanism becomes less and less effective. The reason older people look different from younger ones has to do with oxidative damage in the body's proteins over a lifetime.

Proteins are most responsible for the daily functioning of living organisms. Over the last decade, many researchers have verified that protein modification is a major pathway for aging and degenerative diseases. Glycation, one of the major processes that destroys proteins, occurs when proteins react with sugars. Then, through a series of reactions, including oxidation, advanced glycation end products (the so-called AGEs) form. AGEs accelerate aging processes and promote degenerative disease. This is the equivalent of browning food in the oven—and it is equally irreversible.

Therefore, if we can reduce our rate of living, i.e., metabolic rate, we can extend our productive life and maximum lifespan.

3.2   MAMMALS' CALORIES PER BODY WEIGHT

Science has discovered that the higher the metabolic rate, the lower the maximum life span among mammals. *The Biology of Aging,* edited by J.A. Behnke, et al., 1978, reported research by Richard G. Culter demonstrating the relationship between maximum life-span potential and specific metabolic rate for some common mammals, as shown in the following diagram.

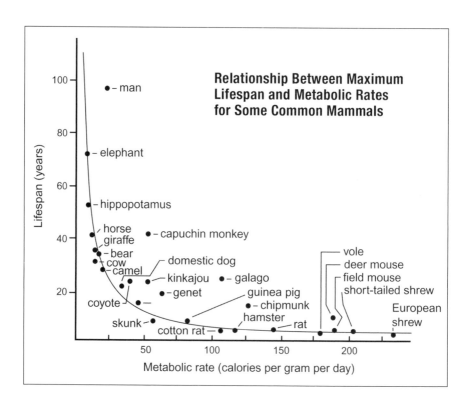

For example, a dog has a maximum life-span potential of about one-sixth the human life expectancy.

Non-mammals have a similar phenomenon between life span and metabolic rate. A well-known scientific study on worms, published in the *Proceedings of the National Academy of Sciences of the United States of America* in 1999, shows that longevity is increased when the metabolic rate goes down and vice versa. Mutations of the soil worm that increase its longevity could define which specific genes are involved in the aging process. The actions from these gene mutations could reduce animal metabolic rate and, consequently, increase longevity. Environmental conditions that reduce the worm's metabolic rate also extend longevity. It was found that the metabolic rate of long-lived mutations is reduced compared with that of worms found in the wild. However, when a certain gene was "turned off," it restored normal longevity and higher metabolic rate to the long-lived mutants. Thus the increased longevity may result from lowering their metabolic rate rather than an alteration of a genetic pathway that leads to enhanced longevity.

The freshwater pearl mussel (*margaritifera margaritifera*), another non-mammalian example, with a life span of over 150 years in polar climates, is one of the longest-lived animals on earth. An ongoing study of the species is being conducted by scientists at the Institute of Developmental Biology in Moscow in order to generate genetic and physiological mechanisms contributing to longevity.

The study compares six southern populations of pearl mussels in Spain, with maximum-recorded ages of 28–40 years, to three Arctic populations in northwest Russia, with maximum ages of 116–155 years. Within Arctic populations, 20% of mussels live more than 90 years in rivers that are pristine. Possible evolutionary significance of northern longevity is an adaptation to severe cold and unstable environments in high gradient rivers. During winter, mussels have a near famine existence during the Polar Night.

In response, northern populations have much lower metabolic rates, reducing energy expenditure for growth under normal as well as extreme conditions. However, this species is capable of increasing its metabolic rate up to 130 times for tissue regeneration and self-healing.

As we will discuss later in this chapter, caloric restriction is the most effective way of reducing metabolic rate. However, in the modern world, we do the opposite—we dramatically increase our caloric intake and thus our metabolic rate.

In summary: *Vibrant health and long healthy life are associated with a greatly reduced long-term metabolic rate. The most effective way to reduce metabolic rate is to restrict calories.*

3.3   CALORIC RESTRICTION

Caloric restriction without malnutrition is the only scientifically recognized method to expand life. It extends the maximum life span, delays and reduces degenerative diseases and dramatically slows aging.

> "So far, caloric restriction remains the only proven way to extend maximum life span (at least in rodents). It is known to enhance DNA repair and retard the decline of mitochondrial function. What's most important, caloric restriction extends 'health span.' Calorie-restricted animals stay healthy and active almost to the very end, showing much less cardiovascular disease or degenerative brain disease. Caloric restriction has a proven neuroprotective effect, with less neuropathology and more neurogenesis (production of new nerve cells) being found in calorie-restricted animals. The development of cataracts is also delayed. Calorie-restricted animals tend to die a sudden death, without a long period of terminal illness. If these findings apply to humans, they are of profound significance, since quality of life in the older years is a critical issue, not to mention the soaring costs of health care."
>
> —*LIFE EXTENSION MAGAZINE,* JUNE 2002

How does caloric restriction work in the human body? Some scientists believe that caloric restriction likely operates through basic and universal mechanisms having to do with energy utilization. All organisms need energy to survive. Depending on their species, they take energy from many different environmental sources, such as air, water, soil, plants and animals they eat. To be successful in its evolution, each organism must also develop finely tuned responses for gauging the availability of energy to determine how much they should consume, when it should be consumed and what should be stored for later use. Based on patterns of energy consumption, responses are made that determine growth and reproduction as well as further food-seeking behavior.

For many organisms, like *C. elgans*, a kind of worm, expectation of low energy availability, triggered by overpopulation, produces a dormant stage of development called the dauer larva. In this form, the organism is small and reproductively immature, but it can withstand environmental stressors and can live many weeks longer than it typically does. When the energy environment is more favorable, the organism reverts to its normal form and continues to develop and mature and then finally shows signs of aging and dies. There are many invertebrates with similar strategies for dormancy. In mammals, a possible parallel strategy is hibernation.

While caloric restriction does not produce a dauer larva or a formal state of hibernation in mammals, many gerontologists are intrigued by the parallels and the evolutionary significance of this strategy. We can consider that the mammalian response to caloric restriction follows a similar strategy (although it does not go as far as in some species) because of the remarkable parallels between the physiological effects of caloric restriction and those of hibernation, among them reduced blood glucose, insulin and white blood cell counts.

Recent genetic studies have shed light on the possibility that caloric restriction might operate through a pathway similar to that which controls the formation of the dauer larva. Several genes have been identified that promote longevity. When the expression of one of these genes is reduced or mutated, the worm can enter the dauer stage, exhibiting a nearly doubled life span compared to worms with the normal gene.

It may be true that the rate of consumption of our vital essence is proportional to the rate that calories are burned by the body.

Again: Eat less, live longer.

Now let's look at some scientific studies of the wide impact of caloric restriction on our bodies.

3.3.1   Rat Experiments

There are many animal studies showing the effect of caloric restriction on maximum life span. The first report was by Professor Clyde McCay of Cornell University in 1935, showing that animals on calorie-restricted diets far outlived animals allowed to eat as much as they wanted.

Studies on rats conducted by Dr. Roy Walford at the UCLA School of Medicine in 1986 also demonstrated dramatic improvement of life span. Rats have a maximum life span of around 35 months, equivalent to a human's 120 years. Every 10 months of a rat's lifetime is about 34 years of a human life. Experiments have shown that a 10% restriction of calories can delay a rat's aging and maximum life span by 10 months, equivalent to about 34 years in a human. A 50% restriction delays aging by 18 months in rats, equivalent to about 60 years in a human.

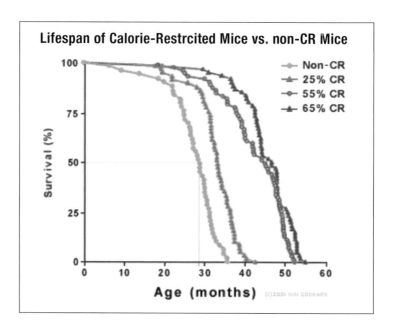

This is increases maximum life span by 50%. Since disease is usually associated with aging, a delay of aging by 50% is an extension of healthy, youthful life.

3.3.2 Monkey Experiments

Monkeys resemble humans more than rats do but are difficult to study because of their longer life span. A long-term groundbreaking primate study is being conducted by a team of scientists led by Dr. R. Weindruch at the University of Wisconsin-Madison. A preliminary report was published by Jennifer Christensen and Richard Weindruch, "Calorie Restriction in Monkeys" in *Life Extension*, July 1998.

Monkey experiments show that a 26% reduction in calorie intake can result in 0.5°F reduction in body temperature, 28% reduction in glucose, 77% reduction in insulin, 30% reduction in weight, 66% reduction in body fat and 400% increase in insulin sensitivity. High insulin sensitivity is a sign of high metabolic efficiency—similar to a highly efficient car engine.

The data is summarized in the following table:

MONKEY EXPERIMENT ON CALORIC RESTRICTION	
NORMAL DIET	REDUCED DIET
Food intake daily: 662 calories	Food intake daily: 488 calories
Body weight: 31.5 pounds	Body weight: 20.5 pounds
Body fat: 26%	Body fat: 8.6%
Abdominal measure: 24.4 inches	Abdominal measure: 16.5 inches
Body mass: 47.6 (kg/m^2)	Body mass: 34.2 (kg/m^2)
Basal glucose: 74	Basal glucose: 53
Basal insulin: 44	Basal insulin: 10
Insulin sensitivity: 1.8 (x10^{-4})	Insulin Sensitivity: 9.1 (x10^{-4})
Leptin: 5.8 (ng/milliliter)	Leptin: 1.0 (ng/milliliter)

3.3.3   Human Experiments

Human experiments are even more difficult. In 1988, the first man-made full biosphere project was conducted in Tucson, Arizona, with eight people enclosed in a sealed environment. They lived with their own air, plants, environment, animals and natural resources without outside help. The eight scientists participated in a caloric restriction program for the next six months, eating an 1800 calorie per day whole food diet (compared with an average 2500 calorie American diet). The results were published by Waldord et al, in the *Proceedings of the National Academy of Sciences*, 1992, a remarkable improvement in health:

- 15% reduction of weight

- 24% lower blood sugar

- 38% lower cholesterol

- 30% reduction of blood pressure

- 27% reduction of white blood cell count

BIOSPHERE 2 EXPERIMENT							
(on eight Biospherans before and after 6 months)							
	BODY WEIGHT		BLOOD SUGAR		CHOLESTEROL		BLOOD PRESSURE	
	BEFORE	AFTER	BEFORE	AFTER	BEFORE	AFTER	BEFORE	AFTER
1	208	158	105	82	215	129	100/70	80/50
2	148	135	81	77	145	100	100/70	90/60
3	148	126	89	60	196	107	110/72	70/40
4	150	127	99	72	190	125	135/90	110/70
5	165	142	101	69	209	122	110/80	100/60
6	130	115	77	68	146	83	100/60	80/40
7	123	111	101	68	231	168	110/80	90/60
8	116	100	80	73	199	119	110/70	85/50
Average	148	126	92	70	191	119	109/77	76/57
Change		15%		24%		38%		30/27%

3.3.4   Effect on Cancer

Cancer is the result of an accumulation of toxins, oxidation of body systems and degeneration of energy potential. Caloric restriction is proven to delay aging, extend maximum life span and thus greatly reduce the risk of cancer. A few experiments performed on rats at the UCLA School of Medicine have shown the incidence of various spontaneous cancers in mice on a calorie-restricted diet compared with normally fed mice.

EFFECT OF CALORIC RESTRICTION ON CANCER IN MICE		
CANCER	% IN NORMAL FED	% IN RESTRICTED FED
Breast	40%	2%
Lung	60%	30%
Leukemia	65%	10%
Liver	64%	11%

The calorie-restricted group also had cancer 8 to 12 months later than the normal fed group. This is equivalent to 15 to 30 years of a human's life. Extending youthful life by 15 to 30 years is a wonderful thing for anyone.

3.3.5   Effect on Brain Body Ratio

The life span of many mammalian species is related to the average weight of the adult brain and the average weight of the adult body, a relationship called the index of cephalization. The heavier the brain, as compared to the body weight, the more long-lived a species will be. This relationship, first reported in 1910, was independently rediscovered in 1955 and refined for mammals by the late gerontologist George Sacher.

Experiments have compared farm-raised rats, which were normally fed, to wild rats, which went through fast and feast in the wilderness. It took the farm rats 70 days to reach a body weight of 270g, at which point their brains each weighed 1.7g. However, it took the wild rats 318 days to reach 270g with brain weights of 2.3g. This is a four-times slower aging rate and 35% larger brain for the same body size, showing the important benefit of caloric restriction.

3.3.6   Effect on Hormones

As will be discussed in Chapter 7, most hormones decline and become imbalanced as we age. This is a fundamental cause of many degenerative diseases. Thus maintaining a youthful hormone system is critically important. Caloric restriction is one of the best methods to naturally maintain youthful hormones longer without hormone replacement.

Taking testosterone as an example, scientists have published several reports showing the effect of caloric restriction on rats. Male rats were divided into two control groups, one with 50% caloric restriction and the other with normal food intake. Results are shown in the graph below.

Rats in the calorie-restricted group showed a 20-day delay

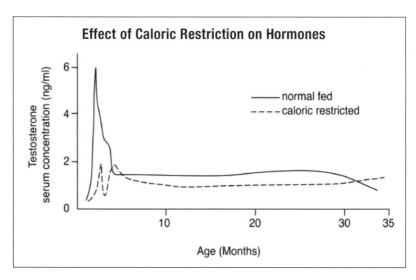

Merry, B.J., & Holehan, A.M., "Serum profiles of LH, FSH, testosterone and 5-alpha-DHT from 21 to 1000 days of age in ad libitum fed and dietary restricted rats," *Experimental Gerontology,* 16: 431, 1981

(equivalent to $2^1/_2$ human years) in pubertal peak of serum testosterone, a 30% lower testosterone level at the peak, and constant testosterone levels throughout life as opposed to the normally fed group's hormone levels declining with age.

The meaning of the chart is significant. Not only is maturity delayed (and thus according to the law of living, aging is delayed), but also active sex life and other benefits of testosterone are extended.

3.3.7 Effect on Athletic Performance

Among other benefits of caloric restriction are athletic performance and immune function. Normally fed and calorie-restricted mice were given a logrolling test. Mice in the calorie-restricted group at age 32 months (about 100 years for a human) could perform logrolling as if they were 12 months old (equivalent to a human's 35). However the normal fed group of 32-month old mice fell off the roller almost every time.

3.3.8 Effect on Immune Function

Many scientific experiments have proved that caloric restriction increases immune system capability. Studies have shown caloric restriction improves immune function in rats. Research on rhesus monkeys showed that limiting consumption of calories seems to boost key infection-fighting cells in the immune system.

> "The key finding is that in a primate species, which is very similar to ourselves, there is a very remarkable effect on the maintenance of the immune system with caloric restriction. As people age, changes in the immune system dramatically increase susceptibility to infectious diseases. So-called T cells, which make up an important component of the immune response, appear to be the part of the immune system most affected by aging,"
>
> —DR. JANKO NIKOLICH-ZUGICH, OREGON HEALTH & SCIENCE UNIVERSITY'S VACCINE AND GENE THERAPY INSTITUTE

3.3.9   Effect on Free Radicals

Studies, such as the one led by Dr. Ricardo Gredilla of Complutense University, published in *The FASEB Journal*, titled "Caloric restriction decreases mitochondrial free-radical generation at complex I and lowers oxidative damage to mitochondrial DNA in the rat heart," have demonstrated that a 40% caloric restriction can lower oxidative damage to mitochondrial DNA by as much as 30%.

According to the free radical theory, aging is due to lifelong free radical damages. Evidence of increased free radical activity and aging comes from the observation that larger animals consume less oxygen per unit of body mass than do smaller animals and they exhibit a correspondingly longer lifespan.

Similarly, cold-blooded animals are more resistant to oxidative stress when maintaining a lower body temperature.

Presumably, lower metabolic activity produces fewer free radicals. Decreasing the flying activity of drosophilae (fruit flies) by wing clipping or space restriction markedly increases survival time. Similarly, queen bees, which do not fly, live approximately 50 times longer than the worker bees that do.

3.3.10   Effect on Heart

Investigators at Washington University School of Medicine in St. Louis studied heart function in members of an organization called the Caloric Restriction Society. They found the calorie-restrictors' hearts were able to relax between beats in a manner similar to the way hearts behave in younger people. Ultrasound examinations showed that the hearts appeared more elastic than those of age- and gender-matched control subjects. This is the first study to demonstrate that long-term caloric restriction with optimal nutrition has cardiac-specific effects that ameliorate age-associated declines in heart function.

3.3.11 Effect on Appearance

A monkey longevity study, published in *Science,* July 2009, showed that 20 years after the experiment began, the monkeys showed many beneficial signs of caloric restriction, including significantly less diabetes, cancer and heart and brain disease. Data from these studies conducted by a team led by Ricki J. Colman and Richard Weindruch at the University of Wisconsin demonstrate that caloric restriction slows aging in a primate species. Of special interest are photos of the monkeys with and without caloric restriction.

The monkeys in the following pictures are of similar age, Canto, left, a 27-year-old rhesus monkey, is on a restricted diet, while Owen, 29, is not. The two monkeys are part of a study of the links between diet and aging.

Does one of them look dramatically younger than the other?

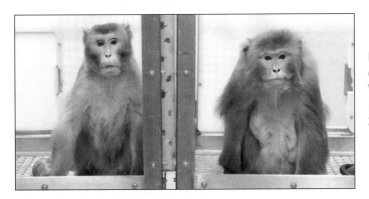

Image courtesy of Dr. Richard Weindruch, et al, *Science,* July 2009.

3.3.12 Effect on Inflammation

Published on the *Journal of Clinical Endocrinology and Metabolism* in 2006, a study led by Dr. Luigi Fontana, at Washington University in St. Louis and the Istituto Superiore di Sanita, Rome, Italy, examined found that caloric restriction (CR) decreases the circulating concentration of a powerful inflammatory molecule called tumor necrosis factor alpha (TNF). They say the combination of lower T3 levels and reduced inflammation may slow the aging process by reducing the body's metabolic rate as well as oxidative damage to cells and tissues.

3.4   IMPLEMENTATION OF CALORIC RESTRICTION

It is without dispute by the scientific community that caloric restriction without malnutrition is the ONLY scientific proven way of extending maximum healthy lifespan. There is overwhelming proof of the benefit to health and longevity as we discussed in Section 3.3. Studies have also shown that you don't have to start at early age to enjoy the benefit.

With such benefit to life, you must be very motivated to undertake a calorie-restricted diet. In this section we discuss the framework of PingLongevity™ Caloric Restriction protocols.

3.4.1   The Difficulty

Even with the overwhelming benefits of caloric restriction, most experts quickly admit that it is very difficult to implement.

> "The huge problem with this proven way to extend maximum life span is human unwillingness to restrict food intake. True, there are drugs that effectively diminish appetite, but this gives rise to questions of side effects and long-term safety. The practical answer might lie in "caloric restriction mimics"—foods made with non-metabolizable ingredients. Such foods can create the feeling of satisfaction while providing only a fraction of the calories. 2-deoxyglucose is a standard caloric restriction mimic used in most studies, but it is unsuitable for human consumption due to toxicity."
>
> —*LIFE EXTENSION MAGAZINE*, JUNE 2002

Here is another quote from an article written by Dr. Stephen Coles of the Los Angeles Gerontology Research Group in 1996:

> "Although the causal relation between caloric restriction and maximum life-span extension was discovered as long ago as 1932, even today, it is still the only known intervention, possibly along with pineal cross transplantation, shown to produce such an effect. Yet no one appears willing to use this method to pro-

long life. Why not? Because people are more interested in the quality of life than in its quantity and the inconvenience factor of always being hungry makes it prohibitive."
—Dr. Stephen Coles

Other experts may even promote a diet with higher caloric intake and metabolism than normal.

"Vegetarians consume the same amount or even significantly more calories than their meat-eating counterparts, and yet are still slimmer . . . What's the secret? One factor that I've mentioned previously is the process of thermogenesis, which refers to our production of body heat during metabolism. Vegetarians have been observed to have a slightly higher rate of metabolism during rest, meaning they burn up slightly more of their ingested calories as body heat rather than depositing them as body fat."
—Prof. Colin Campbell

In the following sections, you will see that with the Ping-Longevity™ Diet, implementing caloric restriction is relatively easy. We do not promote "caloric restriction mimics." We believe it can be implemented naturally and practically since we have helped so many clients and we have seen the results.

3.4.2   Nutrition—the Necessary Condition

You may wonder why in some developing countries, the people who are deprived of food and constantly living in hunger often have short lives. Aren't they on caloric restriction? It is critically important that caloric restriction must be combined with high nutritional density per caloric intake, as we discussed in Section 2.4. This is why in his book, *Beyond the 120 Years Diet,* Dr. Roy Walford calls it CRON (Caloric Restriction with Optimal Nutrition). Other people talk about CRAN (Caloric Restriction with Adequate Nutrition).

What PingLongevity™ Caloric Restriction wants is caloric restriction with the PingLongevity™ Diet, discussed in Chapter 2, which is caloric restriction with PERFECT nutrition.

3.4.3   Use Ideal Weight, Not Calorie Count

Here we are discussing caloric restriction. Exactly how many calories are we talking about? How do we count calories?

How many calories do we need? There are only two tests: Do you keep a constant weight? Do you feel energetic? The intake of calories must be no more than the calories burned. If you take in more calories than you burn, the calories have no place to go but to add to your weight. Therefore, the best measure of caloric intake is your weight.

You don't have to count calories. It should be a closed loop feedback system. You should watch your weight and adjust your calorie intake to keep the weight at the ideal. If you keep the weight at the ideal and make sure of sufficient nutrition, you should always feel energetic. If you lack energy, question your nutritional intake, since we must make sure to restrict caloric intake *without malnutrition.*

What is your ideal body weight? Calorie-counter books will tell you that your ideal weight is your body mass index (BMI), defined as your weight in kilograms divided by the square of your height in meters. They say that if the number is less than 18.5, you are underweight. If it is higher than 25, you are overweight. This is based on statistics of the average population. Nowadays we have many recommended numbers, such as the daily dietary allowance, the normal blood pressure, normal blood sugar levels and ideal weight. However, these are all based on the range of statistical averages. Everyone is genetically different.

A very thin person may be perfectly healthy, but way below the average weight. An average weight would be bad for a naturally thin person because it asks for unnatural weight gain. The other bad thing about average calculations is that usually the optimal figure is at the very low end or high end of the "normal" range. Take blood sugar, for example. The medically recommended blood sugar level is 70–100. If you are 95, you are considered in great shape. However, for what we call *vibrant health,* the super-healthy human, we'd like to see you at 70–85.

In PingLongevity™, we maintain between the ages of 18 and 22, we achieve peak energy, when the body is supposed to be in the best physical shape—either heavy or light, depending on genetic makeup. After this age, energy is moving into the down cycle. The key to vibrant health is to delay and slow the down cycle. It is not difficult to conclude that the ideal weight for most individuals is the weight of the same individual at age 18 to 22.

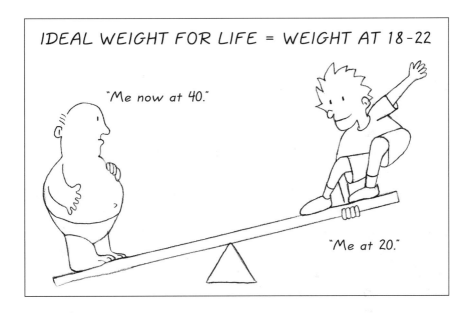

Use your ideal weight as the benchmark. Don't go lower than that. See how much lower calorie intake you can achieve by going for higher quality foods and training the body adapt to lower calories.

3.4.4   Achieving Ideal Weight with Caloric Restriction

The goal of caloric restriction with perfect nutrition is to eat 30 to 50% fewer calories than "normal" (for example, that of what standard BMI formula says), while maintaining as close as possible to ideal weight, with the same lifestyle as "normal" caloric intake.

If you consistently eat a low calorie diet, your body will learn to make your metabolism more efficient, similar to a more efficient engine, which uses less gas for the same mileage. If you continue to reduce your caloric intake, your body will have to lose weight when it reaches maximum metabolic efficiency. At this time, you need to stabilize your caloric intake to maintain the equilibrium. Usually, your body weight at this time will be about the same as when you were 18 to 22 years old.

For example, based on our clinical experience, a person with normal 2200-calorie standard diet can easily take a 1000 to 1200 calorie PingLongevity™ Diet, and be able to sustain an ideal weight.

There are several ways of achieving higher quality of life with caloric restriction:

First, eat high-quality nutritious food to maximize the nutrition value per calorie intake. This way, your intake is more efficient so the body needs fewer total calories. The PingLongevity™ Diet is ideally suited for caloric restriction.

> "Generally speaking, you can eat as much as you want and still lose weight—as long you eat the right type of food."
> —Prof. Colin Campbell

What Prof. Campbell talked about is that if you eat the right type of food, you can lose weight, achieve ideal weight, eat fewer calories and still not feel hungry. There should not be any compromise of enjoyment in life.

Second is to know how to eat quantities of food without consuming too many calories. Here's an experiment: Take a bowl of salad or greens, cook it and see how much is left. Eating a large quantity of raw vegetables equates to a small amount of cooked ones in volume. Now try to eat nuts. A cup of roasted peanuts is approximately 120 calories compared to 250 calories for a medium-sized cone of ice cream or 300 in a single hamburger or 280 in a single chocolate bar. But peanuts will keep you from being hungry much longer because they have a low glycemic index of 14 and are also very high in protein. Another example is raw milk. A cup of raw milk is many times more calorically efficient than a cup of cooked or pasteurized milk. Thus you need fewer calories for the same body needs. By eating more foods like this, you can reduce the number of calories you eat each day.

A third way to reduce calories is to use alternative fuel, such as air, cosmic rays and water, in line with nature's fourth law of food. This requires purifying your spirit and opening up your channels so you can communicate directly with the cosmic energy source.

Fourth, don't burn calories just to be burning them. This is equivalent to burning gas by allowing your car's engine to idle. Extreme exercise wears and tears bones and muscles, accelerates metabolic rate (and the rate of living), and produces no useful work. Light exercise is good without going too far. To reduce weight, the only way is to control caloric input.

Fifth, don't eat if you're not hungry.

> "People often speak of hunger as being a barrier to practicing CRAN, but I think people often eat for reasons other than hunger. People eat out of habit—because it is 'mealtime' (a social ritual). People regularly eat for enjoyment—to entertain themselves (a popular form of recreation). People eat because of appetite—something very distinct from hunger. And people eat until they are 'full.' Eating to satiety is very difficult to avoid, even for me. Resisting the temptation to start eating is much easier than ceasing to eat once eating has begun."
>
> —Ben Best, President, Cryonics Institute

You should not eat if you're not hungry even if it's meal time, unlike many people who have to eat whenever it's time, morning, noon, evening. This way you can cut your caloric intake dramatically. However, if you know you'll have a sport or event coming up that will consume a lot of energy, you should consciously eat a meal a few hours before with a few extra calories and more energy foods. Thus, it is key to understand that caloric restriction means that you want your body to be in a hypo-metabolism state most of the time. Then occasionally whenever you need to perform physically (hyper metabolism), you take in more calories. This is counterintuitive to the fad of increasing your metabolism in order to reduce weight. Be wise to stay young!

If you weigh much more than your ideal weight (your weight at age 18 to 22), reduce calories (and weight) gradually. Burning fat too fast oxidizes the body too quickly. Be persistent and take many small steps over a 6- to 12-month period to get down to the ideal weight. We summarize this section with a story of James:

"I had been slim, muscular, youthful, healthy and energetic until I turned 40. Then I gained 25 pounds in two years. I ate as much as I did when I was in my 20s and often felt tired after a day at work. I developed allergies, coughing, sneezing and a runny nose. I ate mostly Chinese stir-fried food, pork, vegetables, packaged frozen vegetables, tofu, skim milk, thinking I was on a much healthier diet than the usual fast food. But my weight continued to increase and I started to notice my belly. I sometimes stared at old pictures of myself, envying the boyish body and found myself thinking about my overweight father, uncle and grandfather having heart disease, diabetes and high blood pressure.

I didn't move like I did as a kid. I needed to reduce calorie intake, but I got hungry because my body was accustomed to the routine of mealtime. A little further research made me realize that some foods made me hungry the more I ate them, while others made me full for a long time.

Here is the secret: The same quantity of raw food has about twice the volume as when it is cooked. Also, foods like nuts, with a high protein value but very low insulin sensitivity, keep me feeling full for a long time. Lastly, raw food has more nutritional value for the same quantity. I don't need to take in as much raw food as cooked food.

I started changing my routines while still enjoying food and life. In the morning, I drink two glasses of raw milk bought at a whole food store, plus multivitamin and mineral supplements. The multivitamins and minerals are just for insurance purposes because vegetables and fruits may grow in nutritionally depleted soil and fast-raised chickens and cows may not be as nutritious as before. Occasionally, I add a little protein powder, one with digestive enzymes. I drink plenty of green tea (more than 10 cups) throughout the day. I eat a half-cup of roasted peanuts at lunchtime, which stuffs me for the rest of the day.

Six out of seven nights a week, I eat healthy raw deep ocean fish (tuna), shellfish (oysters), fresh seaweeds (from an Oriental grocery store), raw fresh vegetables (seasoned with uncooked apple cider vinegar, unprocessed honey, and raw sea salt), and tofu. I eat very little starchy food (bread, rice). The more I eat this diet, the less I need flavor. Occasionally, I want junk food—mostly Chinese or Italian at social gatherings. When I do eat junk food, I skip meals the next day to let my body cleanse itself. I can enjoy food and life and vibrant health too.

My new eating plan turns out to require less than one-fourth of the calories I had in my 20s. Within a few months, I got back to my young adult figure with muscles and no belly. My allergy is gone. I am as energetic as 20 years ago. I play competitive sports with people in their 20s. My life is vibrant again in my 40s."

—JAMES, SAN DIEGO

3.5 EFFECTIVE WEIGHT CONTROL

The last decades have been dubbed the Fat Decades. In the article, "World's Fattest Countries," *Forbes Magazine* summarized recent statistics:

> "There are currently 1.6 billion overweight adults in the world, according to the World Health Organization. That number is projected to grow by 40% over the next 10 years."
>
> —*FORBES MAGAZINE*

Even in the context of constant warnings from every health organization in the world about our bulging waistlines, the findings are stunning. They come in the face of growing knowledge about the risk of being overweight and a steady stream of public health messages about the benefits of exercise and low-fat diets. And they raise disturbing prospects that the nation faces an ever-increasing prevalence of diabetes, cardiovascular disease and other health problems associated with obesity.

"We don't use the word 'epidemic' lightly," said Jeffrey P. Koplan, former director of the CDC. "This is an unexpected rapid increase in the number of cases of obesity and it's really remarkable. Indeed, the speed of the increase was characteristic not of chronic conditions, but of communicable diseases like the flu."

The increase in obesity was found across age and gender groups and geographic regions, suggesting "that there have been sweeping changes in U.S. society that are contributing to weight gain." The highest increases occurred in people between 18 and 29 years old and in those with at least some college education.

Public health officials measure weight using the body mass index (BMI), defined as the metric weight divided by the square of the metric height. Obesity is defined as a BMI of 30 or over. Generally, people with a BMI of between 25 and 29.9 are considered overweight. A "normal" BMI is 19 to 24.9.

Calorie requirements drop as people age because we aren't growing (unless it's a belly!) anymore and we don't exercise as much. Despite that, our consumption of calories usually does not decrease with age. We tend to eat the same amounts even when we are not really hungry. We still keep a teenager's schedule of three meals and two snacks a day. Thus we consume more calories than we can burn and we put on weight.

Many of us were erroneously led to believe that if we don't eat fat, we won't gain weight. However, all foods—protein, fat and carbohydrates—have their caloric values. If your calorie intake (not just the amount of fat) is more than you need, the food will be converted to fat or semi-digested gunk. There are vegetarians who are overweight because they eat too many calories, although not in meat, more than the body can consume.

When you take in more calories than necessary, there are only a few ways to deal with it. The body has to burn the calories through an equal amount of converted work (exercise, labor). It can also convert the calories into fat to store in the body.

There is a third way to deal with the excess calories. When a person consumes more than necessary and continues to gain weight due to stored fat, the body becomes less efficient, even in making fat. Our weight cannot grow infinitely, so the body starts to store "junk," things that are toxic and foreign. The body also becomes a non-productive machine. It uses enzymes and energy to try to digest food. The semi-digested food is also largely expelled from the body. Thus, you waste energy and enzyme potential on harmful work.

The obese often engage in intensive exercise programs. They hire the best trainers. They sweat, jog, lift weights. They may even burn some fat or consume the extra calories to keep fat constant. But they cannot keep up with the hard regimen and so they put the fat back on.

They then try something different. They grab one of the fad diets and eat powders or pre-packaged meals for a few weeks to lose weight. It works, except it cannot be sustained forever. So they gain the fat back.

Three negative side effects can occur. First, as discussed earlier, fat is a very inefficient fuel source for the body. It generates more byproducts of oxidants, which accelerate aging. As you burn fat, you age faster. Second, you go through fat and lean cycles, and your skin has to adapt to larger or smaller sizes. Your skin loses elasticity after the mid-30s, and you appear older than you are. Third and most importantly, the body simply does not need, nor can it use up, the intake of extra calories.

The fact is, we burn many fewer calories than when we were growing, yet we still keep the habit of eating three meals and two desserts a day and consume the same amount we did when we were youngsters.

In conclusion, storing fat—nature's protection against severe conditions such as freezing temperatures or famine—is unnecessarily used in modern society as a daily endeavor. The body will adapt. If you want your body to simply be a digestion machine, it will. When the body is overfed, like your car's engine, it runs dirtier inside and becomes less efficient.

PingLongevity™ defines the ideal weight to be what you weigh at 18 to 22 years old. It is *your* ideal rather than someone else's ideal average. Any weight over your ideal is due to taking in more calories than you burn.

But how do we lose weight and control weight? Weight control is a very complex issue. It's not simply due to a lack of discipline. It is multi-faceted. That is why so many fad weight loss programs do not work in long term. To be effective in weight loss and control, you must know the root causes and use an effective program to address the issues that led to your excess weight.

You must consider weight control from the following angles:

- **Food intolerance:** As you have learned in Section 2.9, almost everyone has certain silent food allergies. This is due to long term habitual consumption of certain foods. The body develops an immune rejection of these foods. As a result, you cannot absorb these foods, even if they are highly nutritionally dense foods, you cannot absorb them. You constantly need more nutrients and hence a craving for more calories. In our clinical experience, getting rid of food intolerance can mean a significant reduction of unwanted weight.

  "Approximately 90 to 95% of patients in our clinic lose weight after correcting food intolerances. Linda, a 65-year-old patient, has been battling her weight problem all her life and also suffering chronic severe sinus problem. She has tried every method of losing weight with no success, despite an intensive exercise program that includes tennis and cardio exercises six days a week.

  I recommended food allergy test several times before she decided to take my advice. After just three weeks of avoiding foods that tested positive for allergies, Linda came back to thank me, and said, 'Why didn't I do this earlier? You are absolutely right! I don't feel hungry anymore. My blood sugar is stable. With three trips from Seattle to New York and one wedding, I thought I'd gain weight. But actually my weight went from 186 to 175 pounds in just two weeks. I also lost two bra sizes when

I was trying the dress for my girl friend's wedding. I lost especially in the abdominal area, which has been difficult.'

Linda has continued losing weight and her sinus problem has disappeared."

—DR. PING

"Patsy, a 59-year-old patient, a mother of two boys, told me that the beauty of our weight loss program is that she doesn't need to do a lot of exercise.

'After I lost weight, it stayed off and I haven't regained any of it,' Patsy told me.

She lost a total of 37 pounds without adding any exercise or diet pills. Her husband commented about her "returning to teenager's figure," and went to shopping with her to buy new jeans. That was something that had never happened before!

'Dr. Ping, this not only helps my health, builds my confidence, and also strengthens my family relationship.'"

—DR. PING

- **A diet high in calories but low in nutrition:** About 99% of the people we see are on diets without optimal nutrition, regardless of whether they are meat eaters or vegetarians. Empty calories are a large percent of their diets. (Section 2.4.6). When you're on a less than optimal diet, your body will constantly tell you that it needs more nutrients. Therefore, you want more foods, which give you more empty calories. In our clinical experience, once you are on a highly scientific diet, such as the PingLongevity™ Diet, you are so satisfied that you eat far fewer calories. It's the best way to lose and control weight.

- **Acidity:** As discussed in Section 2.3, many of us eat a diet overloaded with acid forming foods. For the body to keep a constant alkalinity in our major fluids such as blood, it has to pull in from our alkaline reserve and to store extra acid in fat. Fat becomes the body's protection mechanism. As a result, if you're eating quantities of acid-forming foods every day, it becomes very difficult to lose fat and body weight. Therefore, it's important for you to switch to alkaline forming foods and drink alkaline water.

- **Insulin resistance:** Most insulin resistance, or sometimes referred to as Metabolic Syndrome and Type 2 diabetes in more severe cases, is due to poor lifestyle choices. Over time, as the body is bombarded with high glycemic index foods and insulin spikes, the body develops insensitivity to insulin, thus lose its ability to burn fat. This is extensively discussed in Section 2.2.

- **Toxicity:** When the body is overloaded with toxins, the immune system is busy. It requires more nutrients, thus more food and more calories. Therefore, for any weight loss and control program, detoxification is very important. You should use the program outlined in Section 2.10 to periodically detoxify all of your body systems.

- **Sex hormone imbalance:** As it will be discussed in Chapter 7, hormone imbalance can have huge implication in your weight control. For example, if you are estrogen dominant (Section 7.2.5) in both men and women, you'll experience weight gain and it will be difficult to lose weight.

- **Thyroid hormone imbalance:** We have seen many people who are iodine deficient, which causes thyroid hormone imbalance (Section 7.2.2). You may have hypothyroidism, namely too low a metabolism to control your weight.

- **Stress:** Stress has a really significant impact on weight control, as will be discussed in Section 7.2.3. You must manage your modern day stress effectively. Follow the protocols in Chapter 6.

- **Liver impairment:** In our clinic, we have seen many people who have stagnated liver function. Since the liver is the main organ for producing energy, metabolizing proteins and controlling hormonal balance, an impaired liver will result in a lack of energy and a craving for more food. Thus, detoxifying (Section 2.10) and protecting your liver by staying away from alcohol is very important.

Finally, we have to mention the recent trend of using carbohydrate and fat blockers as effective ways to lose weight. These have been promoted by many health authorities. We are generally against such an approach. One has to wonder, "If you don't want the body to absorb these nutrients, why consume them in the first place? Even if you can effectively block the digestion of these foods, how do you know the body will not store the poorly digested foods elsewhere, leading to increased acidity and toxins in the body?"

3.6 ADULT ONSET DIABETES

It would be interesting to examine the process of adult-onset diabetes because it is almost always an amplified case of the overconsumption of calories. Also called Type 2 diabetes, this is a degenerative disease that is rapidly growing in industrialized countries.

Food is converted into blood sugar. The purpose of insulin is to keep the sugar in the blood at normal levels. Soon after we eat, our blood sugar levels naturally rise. In response, the pancreas releases insulin. As insulin binds to the cells' receptors, it allows sugar to pass from the bloodstream into the body's cells to be used as fuel. Extra blood sugar is converted into fat. In the case of adult-onset diabetes, although the pancreas may produce insulin, the body is insensitive to the insulin action, thus keeping a high blood sugar level.

When blood sugar remains constantly high, the blood becomes thicker, stickier and less fluid. Just think about pure water as compared with sugary water. It is more difficult for thicker blood to travel through small blood vessels, such as those in the eyes and the extremities. When these areas cannot be nourished and toxins cannot be carried away by the blood, functional failures result. For example, that is why diabetics may have eye problems. In addition, thicker blood becomes sticky, depositing itself on the walls of blood vessels. It builds up, narrows the pathways and pollutes the blood circulation system.

A high blood sugar level also causes protein-glucose complexes—medically called AGEs (advanced glycation endproducts) —a form of cellular garbage that accumulates with age and interferes with the workings of the cells. Excess glucose in the blood cross-links with and damages proteins. As more and more proteins are damaged, the body gets old.

Adult-onset diabetes often goes hand-in-hand with being overweight. Besides genetic reasons (which can play an important role, but are not the whole picture), it starts with overeating. When we constantly eat too much over a long period of time, the body has to produce more insulin and bind it to the cells. A constantly high insulin level not only depletes the body's reserve to produce insulin hormones but also makes the cells' receptors less sensitive and efficient. Thus, people become overweight and diabetic.

If diabetes that is caused by excessive caloric intake is an example of accelerated aging, caloric restriction is a great way to decelerate aging. As you can see, the real issue has to do with our choice of lifestyle. One is the accelerated rate of living in which we age much faster and get into the age-related degenerative diseases earlier. The other is a decelerated rate of living. It is our choice indeed.

Most Type 2 diabetes can be effectively corrected through lifestyle. If you follow the protocols outlined in Chapters 2 and 3, you will most likely be able to dramatically lessen and even heal your adult onset diabetes.

3.7   CAN WE LIVE ON LIGHT?

There have been many stories about Chinese Taoist sages who live deep in the sacred mountains. They perform Taoist alchemy every day. They live on the fresh air, high-energy water and the cosmic rays while eating very little food. It was said the ancient sages lived a life of 400 to 1000 years.

In our universe, there are many forms of energy, as will be discussed extensively in Chapter 10. We humans are only able to absorb and digest certain types of energy, mostly in the foods we eat. However, digesting food requires burning more of our life candle because it consumes calories through metabolism as we have discussed in previous sections.

Live food has less energy than direct cosmic energy, such as sunlight, moonlight, high-energy air, high-energy water and the infinite energy of the universe. Most of us have not developed the ability to directly absorb such energies fully, but the more we are able to do so, the less we need to depend solely on food for our energy needs.

Most people have to depend totally on physical food because they do not have the ability to absorb cosmic energy. However, more highly developed beings can partially or completely depend on water, air and cosmic energy (rays). Not only is this a much more efficient use of energy, thus extending life, but the higher frequency energy can also enhance our lives in other ways.

Evidence has shown that it's entirely possible to train our bodies to absorb cosmic energies to reduce our consumption in food calories. This way, we'll live much longer and be vibrantly healthy.

In the book *Life from Light*, Michael Werner and Thomas Stockli documented real experiences of people living without eating. There are real people who lived without food for four years because they could live on the subtle energies from the universe. It's a way to have the body create a near-death experience so that the focus becomes internal. The case studies show many diseases were healed through this process. We cite this without endorsing the method because we believe the method requires further scientific study. In particular, we don't believe one can easily develop a healthy way of absorbing higher energies than foods without a systematic method of alchemy, such as Taoist alchemy as discussed in later chapters.

In China, there is a form of Taoist healing in which people meditate while hiking, but do not sleep for three days. It is similar to creating a near-death experience. With that, many people can heal their illnesses.

In a sense, PingLongevity™ offers a way of *living on light without hardship.* We have so many examples among our patients. For example, people with a normal BMR requirement of 2300 calories a day live on only 1000 to 1200 calories a day. They have much better nutritional status because they use the PingLongevity™ Diet, and kept their weight the same as when they were 18, so they live a vibrant healthy life.

There is a law of thermodynamics that says you must balance the energy you take with the energy you expend to keep your weight constant. Then why are some people able to reduce their energy intake by about 50% without losing weight? There are several possible explanations for this. By practicing PingLongevity™, either:

1. They're partially living on light (which is the best energy form), or

2. They have much more efficient metabolism (i.e., in my car example, a more efficient engine to convert a higher percentage of energy intake to work), or

3. They somehow are able to lower their basal metabolic rate—thus expending less energy.

Whatever is the case, PingLongevity™ process has the potential to create a significantly slower rate of aging—staying young for much longer!

In the coming chapters, we will introduce methods of alchemy that can purify and refine your energy so that you can learn to absorb more energy directly from universal sources of energy, such as sunlight and pure air and reduce the quantity of calories you take in.

3.8   SUMMARY

In this chapter, we discussed caloric restriction, the most exciting and the only scientifically proven way of extending maximum lifespan. The following provides a brief summary:

• Caloric restriction has been scientifically shown to have the potential to extend maximum lifespan, thus productive lifespan, by at least 50% and to slow down the rate of aging by half.

- Caloric restriction has been shown to have dramatic, wide ranging health benefits in all aspects of body systems and in degenerative disease prevention.

- Practicing caloric restriction has been conventionally thought to be impossible. However, PingLongevity™ Caloric Restriction provides a practical way of making the metabolism very efficient.

- Weight loss and weight control require a multi-model approach. That is why so many weight loss programs fail in the long term. You must understand the root cause and use a systematic approach.

Longevity Exercise

The goal of PingLongevity™ Exercise is to retain the ability to remain fully functional for your entire life. We also refer to this method of exercise and fitness as functional fitness. It should include both exercises and protective measures. It not only extends functionality, but also reduces wear and tear on the body. It should include exercises for flexibility, cardiovascular and respiratory functions, resistance and rehabilitation of weak and injured parts of the body. It should also include the entire body mechanics, including the heart, lung, brain, eyes, ears and all groups of muscles, tendons and bones.

"The real science of exercise is to maintain all the necessary body functionality while creating minimum wear and tear."
—DR. TAICHI TZU

The goal of training an athelete is to dramatically increase his competitive performance, sometimes at the cost of wear and tear and injuries to the musculoskeletal system.

The purpose of recreational sports is to have fun, sometimes with negative effects on the body. For example, continuing exposure to sunlight can create long-term damage to the skin.

Most people go the gym to burn calories. We frequently give you the car analogy: It is as though you have to burn a certain number of gallons of gas each day even though you truly don't need to go that many miles. You're running your car aimlessly just to get rid of some gas in your tank. You end up creating a lot more oxidation inside the car and creating needless wear and tear on all systems in the car. Instead, we must deal with weight control and caloric issues differently by using methods we discussed in Chapters 2 and 3.

The purpose of longevity exercises, or PingLongevity™ Exercise is to extend the function of our bodies' mechanical systems for as long as possible. For example, we want our heart muscles to stay strong, eye muscles to be elastic (so we don't need reading glasses), bone density in good condition, spine flexible enough to be able to bent over to tie shoes, arms able to lift weights, strong lung capacity and the brain alert and functional, memory intact.

> "Here, what we teach is flexibility, stability which is your balance, strength and power which is your ability to move weights quickly and move fast, which is what you need to do occasionally in life. So, to function, you have to pick things that resemble what you do in real life. You have to squat, lunge, bend, twist, push and pull. Every day you do a form of that. So I think it's important to do exercises that get you to practice those movements. When you get into the real world, you can get out of your car, you can pick your kids up, you can carry groceries, you can bend over and reach over your head. It's all these movement patterns that are very important to incorporate into your exercises."
>
> —GORDON DUFFY, PRESIDENT, DUFFY FITNESS INSTITUTE

4.1   WHAT'S WRONG WITH MOST EXERCISE?

You have your choice of any type of exerciese you like, whether you engage in competitive sports with a goal of winning trophies or your exercise is recreational goal is simply to have fun. Life is full of compromise. However, if your purpose in exercising is to function like a young person when you're in middle age or even old age, you need to be aware of the pitfalls of many training methods.

4.1.1 The Bias of Sports

Each sport has its own pitfalls. Usually it is biased to a particular group of muscles.

> "Take downhill skiing, for example. The quads are a key muscle group for high performance in these events, so exercises such as leg presses could be considered effective "sport-specific" exercises for downhill skiers. However, if a skier's hamstrings are weak relative to the quads—a common condition with these athletes because downhill skiing places tremendous stress on the quads—the knees are more susceptible to injury. In effect, such an athlete has what I refer to as a structural imbalance.
>
> According to a recent study presented in *IDEA* magazine, the average female aerobics instructor has 18% body fat. This is higher than the average female competitive weightlifter (16%).
>
> According to a recent study published in *Muscular Development* magazine, muscle necrosis (tissue death) and inflammation can be observed in the calves of marathon runners 7 days after a race."
>
> —GORDON DUFFY, PRESIDENT, DUFFY FITNESS INSTITUTE

> "Elite tennis players in their teens appear to have a very high rate of lower spine injury, a new study suggests. Although the subjects in this study did not have symptoms, the researchers point out that these injuries will probably progress to more serious conditions if training techniques are not modified.
>
> The British researchers found that of 33 elite-level tennis players they examined, 85 percent had some sort of abnormality in the lower spine. Damage to the joints at the back of the spine, stress fractures and herniated discs were among the problems seen on MRI scans."
>
> —*REUTERS HEALTH*, JULY 24, 2007

We can talk about many other sports. For example, baseball and softball tend to injure shoulders, elbows, backs, knees, wrists and hands. Golf tends to injure shoulders, backs, elbows, wrists and hands.

Just take a look at the evaluation process used by life insurance companies. Insurance companies make serious money by betting on life expectancy. They hire high-powered statisticians to estimate premiums based on the risk of each individual—how he/she will fare according to age, race, health, occupation, family history and health habits. Professional athletes fall into the high-risk category and command higher premiums for life insurance. According to the American Academy of Orthopedic Surgeons, there were more than three million sports injuries in 1999. A new study at the Duke University Medical Center scanned the knees of 11 basketball players at Duke at the beginning and end of the 1999–2000 season. The magnetic resonance imaging (MRI) snapshots of the knees showed that nearly all of the players had signs of stress, nine out of 22 knees had abnormalities and possible thinning of the cartilage coating the knee bones and three had jumper's knee, which occurs when the tendon connecting the patella to the tibia, or shinbone, gets inflamed. In some cases, it can degenerate and become disabling.

The point here is that participating in one or two types of sports cannot replace longevity exercises. Sports are basically competition based on a set of rules. Sports are not exercise systems designed to promote optimal body function for longevity. Participating in competitive sports may even accelerate wear and tear on the body's mechanical system.

4.1.2   The Bias of Gym Training

If you run for 30 minutes a day, walk on the treadmill every morning, take an aerobics class twice a week, you will miss a lot! Why?

Here is what the renowned fitness expert Gordon Duffy had to say about the pitfalls some of the most widely used fitness exercises such as lifting weights, walking or running on a treadmill, running, sit-ups and aerobics, during an interview by Dr. Taichi Tzu.

> "I want you to get off those treadmills! Stop those aerobics classes! Stop doing sit-ups and please, stop running around the

block! Why, because those activities have no scientific basis for achieving the results you are after and they will not work long term! In fact, they could very well be damaging your health.

The first thing you need to do is fix your imbalances. You need to lift weights to correct your imbalances. For example, if you stand straight and look in the mirror, I bet you are leaning forward, like almost everyone. So exercises like sit-ups that may cause you to lean forward even more, wouldn't be your best choice. So you have to address the body to get it straight. You have to do weight resistance to strengthen the muscles so just from a postural point of view you can stand up straight. If you don't strengthen your lower back and if you don't strengthen your upper back, you'll chronically lean forward and you'll eventually have back problems. In terms of exercise, most of us choose cardio as our first choice. Cardio is a good choice because you need to strengthen your heart. But you need to do the right cardio.

Now you mentioned treadmills. Treadmills are not very effective, because the way you walk on a treadmill is not a normal walking movement. When you walk outside, you're actually walking across the pavement, so you are actually doing what we call "close chain action." You're actually moving your feet one after another and moving your body across the path. When you're on the treadmill, the belt is driving underneath your feet. So you're not going technically over the pavement, you're actually driving the belt underneath you. So what happens is that your hamstrings, your thigh and butt muscles nearly shut down after a while. Yes, your quadriceps and thighs are working, but that puts tremendous stress on your knees. And not only will treadmill walking hurt your knees eventually, since it's not a normal way of walking, it will cause oxidative stress on your brain. Over a period of time, it can negatively affect your thinking process and cognition. So stay away from treadmills and stairmasters.

We suggest you go outside to walk and if you're able to run, try to run shorter distances at the beginning. Do some sprint work. Most important, work on strength training from the beginning to strengthen your body overall and increase body tolerance for weight-bearing exercise.

There's nothing wrong with running for a half hour a day, if you body can tolerate it. You know, it's a pretty significant amount of time. Running will help improve your heart, lymphatic system and nearly all body systems. However, running, especially anything longer than about 400 meters, doesn't develop muscles. Over time, you may improve your heart function to a certain extent with running, but you're going to burn up your muscle. So if you burn up your muscle tissue, that means you'll lose some structural support. The farther you run, the more muscle you burn.

Take a look at Olympic athletes. Sprinters have more muscle; marathoners have less muscle. Who is healthier? That is a subject open to debate. But sprinters usually are very healthy and they carry a lot of muscle, so their bodies are very functional. On the other hand, some marathoners who come to my clinic are actually less fit. If I give them a pair of 20-pound weights and have them walk up and down a few flights of stairs, they are absolutely exhausted.

So what's going to help you in real life? If you need to carry bags of groceries up a couple of flights of stairs into your house, you're going to be best off with weight resistance and sprint training as opposed to long distance running. Running per se is not bad. It's not going to be bad for you, but you must incorporate strength training, short-burst-of-energy types of exercises and other methods to complement running. There's no question about it.

On my radio show, when I advised people to avoid sit-ups, I got a flood of phone calls from angry listeners. Think about it: If you took a string of some sort, whatever you have in your house, you hang it from the ceiling, then stand sideways on it, lining up your ankles, hips and shoulders, most of you will find you are leaning forward. Our lifestyle of sitting at computer keyboards, sitting for long periods of time and even the effects of gravity will pull us forward. Women's breasts and men's larger heads propel us forward and cause us to hunch over. So if you think about it, doing a sit-up will shorten your stomach muscles because you are being pulled forward, exaggerating the problem. Most people do not know how to do sit-ups correctly, so they actually shorten the abdominal muscles. Instead, what you want to do is strengthen the abdominals without pulling you forward. If you strengthen the back muscles, you'll be able to stand taller.

We have all been sold a bill of goods from infomercials that capitalize on our weaknesses. We were once told that running was the way, then sit-ups to give us "six-pack abs." The '80s broke open the aerobic myth and so on. What happened was that there was a huge influx of people trying to get in shape and our system simplified it by creating so-called cure-alls. We are all different, so what makes anyone think that we can all train the same and have the same results?

Guess what? Running, particularly longer distance running can be counterproductive to your goals. It's funny that sprinters who run only 100 meters have less fat and more muscle than the long distance ones. Hmmmmmmmm. We know that nutrition is more important in reducing body fat in the abdominals than doing sit-ups, which actually cause more back issues than I can count. Finally aerobics is a fraudulent system that peaks out over 4 to 6 weeks. The body adapts to the protocol and actually stores fat after that. I have treated several women that came to me with orthopedic issues that arose from aerobic training."

—GORDON DUFFY, PRESIDENT, DUFFY FITNESS INSTITUTE

4.1.3   Exercise to Burn Calories?

Weight management is a complex topic as we have discussed in Section 3.5. The purpose of exercise should not be to burn fat or calories.

Most of the fashionable exercise programs and diet plans promote the idea of that exercise increases calorie burn. But there are several problems with this idea:

First, it promotes the idea of "eating more" and "burning more," which accelerates aging due to unnecessary caloric consumption (see Chapter 3).

Second, it is not an efficient way of losing weight or burning fat. It is very difficult to burn as many calories as most of us, considering our modern lifestyle. In order to burn 100 calories, you need to do any of the following exercises:

- Bicycle riding: 10 minutes
- Walking: 15–20 minutes
- Dancing: 20 minutes
- Tennis: 20 minutes
- Yoga: 20 minutes
- Playing Frisbee: 20–30 minutes

- Swimming: 15 minutes
- Volleyball: 30 minutes
- Skateboarding: 20 minutes
- Kayaking: 20 minutes
- Golfing: 20–30 minutes
- Horseback riding: 20–30 minutes

Well, how easy is it to consume 100 calories? Here are a couple of eye-opening facts about calories:

- One chocolate bar: 200–250 calories
- One Big Mac: 576 calories

- Two slices pepperoni pizza: 406 calories
- One cup of ice cream: 320 calories

You may take in approximately 2500 calories a day. About 75% of those calories are burned for basal metabolic purposes to help sustain bodily functions and life, you are still left an excess of 600 to 700 calories you must burn every day to avoid gaining weight. This requires a lot of "exercises" for a modern white-collar worker!

Many of us, at middle age, go to the gym to beef up our muscles especially the ever-problematic abs, in an effort to look younger and leaner. Yet, even the hardest training might result in well-sculpted muscles everywhere but where you want them and with those stubborn love handles persisting around the waist. It's easy to tell that's a middle-aged hard-trained body! But have you ever thought about young people in their late teens? Why can the boys keep those small waists and the girls those slim hips without hard muscle training in the gym? To keep a young smooth body, you must have 1) a youthful hormone balance resembling that of your 18- to 22-year-old body, and 2) keep your weight at that of your 18- to 22-year-old self so that you don't have more extra fat than fits your genetic type.

"Some of these exercises may be effective ways to lose weight. However, the weight is fat, connective tissue and muscle. So the key is to lose body fat, not weight. That's the real secret. The best way to determine that is your clothing. I have people who come in, saying 'Hey, my clothing fits differently.' One woman who worked here lost $2^1/_2$ pant sizes in 60 days but did not lose one pound, because she kept her muscle. So it's more effective to lose body fat. But the concept of "weight loss" from most therapists' point of view, is not an effective way of describing it. If you lost your puppy, you'll go find your puppy. So if you lose your weight, the tendency subconsciously is to go out to get that weight back. So the best way to describe it, in my opinion, is to say we want to eliminate body fat. Most exercises eliminate some fat, but they also cause muscle loss.

You're probably familiar with the popular television show, "The Biggest Loser." You'll see contestants lose 100 pounds, 150 pounds, but if you look at them closely, how much body fat have they lost? What they lose is water, muscle and fat. They lose everything. The exercise they choose isn't effective in burning just body fat. You don't want to lose muscle, Hours on treadmills and hours of aerobics will fail after a year or two. These people will gain their weight back because they lost the muscle. If you have muscle, you have a metabolic rate like a little metabolic furnace so that you can continue to burn fat. So the exercise you choose as you've seen on these television shows may cause short term success, but long term failure because people cannot exercise 5 to 6 hours a day to keep it off."

—GORDON DUFFY, PRESIDENT, DUFFY FITNESS INSTITUTE

Burning fat itself is not a fun activity. How many times do we hear co-workers, friends, and relatives complain about how difficult exercise is? If exercise is fun, why do we watch TV while doing it? Most of us want to stay fit. The question, then, is why do we get unfit in the first place?

The old saying is true: Work hard, die young. We often get trapped in a dilemma. We know hard labor reduces life span. Yet we put our bodies, especially our digestive systems and metabolic processes, through hard work whenever we put on weight; then we work even harder to take the fat off through strenuous exercise, weight lifting, treadmills and marathons.

In fact, the more we sweat, the faster our hearts pump and the harder we work our muscles, the better we think we're doing. This whole cycle is promoted by fashionable fitness programs that push new equipment, electrical stimulation of muscles, supplements to enhance muscle growth and personal trainers. It has been a passion as well as a fashion. Still, we witness more obesity and more and more pain! It's time to sit back and think through what we are doing to ourselves.

Let's look to nature for answers. In nature, animals labor to make a living (food and shelter), survive predators and have playful fun. Otherwise, they usually lie down, rest, and sleep. Just observe your own pets.

For us, fortunately there is much less need to do hard labor. We have machines. We don't need to run away from predators because we are usually well protected. We have fun playing basketball, golf and tennis. However, we also perform boring tasks for no useful work or fun: lifting weights and walking treadmills. What is the purpose? We are driven to this because we eat too much and need to burn fat. The fat collects under our skin and wraps our organs so we cannot see the beautiful muscle curves of the natural body. Why create the situation in the first place by eating too much—then harm ourselves again by wearing out our mechanical systems through over-exercising?

4.1.4   Wear and Tear on Body Systems

Admittedly, there are many benefits of exercise. It increases blood circulation, raises the levels of HDL (good cholesterol), lowers blood pressure, improves the immune system and helps protect the body against many diseases. It reduces the chance of cardiovascular diseases. According to a famous study of 17,000 male alumni of Harvard University between the ages of 35 and 74, those who actively exercised lowered their overall death rates by 25 to 33% and decreased their risk of coronary artery disease by an astounding 41% when compared with their more inactive fellow alumni. This is easy for us to accept. In fact, it has become fashionable to go to the gym, to hire a personal trainer and to use exercise to burn fat.

Despite the many benefits, most exercises as discussed in the previous sections, create wear and tear, as well as overstressing a few particular areas of the body, potentially causing permanent damage, which could be counter to our purpose of extending youthful functionality to advanced ages.

Like brain cells, muscle cells do not regenerate. Once a muscle cell dies, it cannot be replaced. These cells are different from skin cells. Once a muscle has been subjected to the stress of misuse or overuse, it cannot repair itself. But like brain cells, muscle cells occasionally are capable of changing function to take over the work of nearby damaged cells. In this way, a person is able to continue walking, running, dancing and moving, even though some muscle cells might have been damaged over time. Therefore, we have to be extremely careful not to damage our muscles.

How about building muscle? We all want to look good, have the right amount of muscle and the right body lines. Bodybuilding is most effective when we are very young. Studies have shown a two-fold increase in oxygen metabolism to the muscles during exercise after a brief training session. But while anyone, at any age, can develop stronger and more efficient muscles as a result of exercise training, such conditioning is best begun early in life. The younger you are, the more "trainable" your muscles are. Many forces are at work to determine body shape.

Once muscles are built, they will not be lost until old age, a time when your hormone levels are dramatically reduced or unbalanced, or you are severely deprived of nutrition and caloric intake for a period of time, in which case, exercise won't increase your muscle mass anyway. Losing muscle in middle age is a misconception. It is mainly due to the added fat, which covers all the body lines and muscles. The underlying muscles are still there.

On the other hand, after middle age, trying to increase muscle mass is difficult and can actually creates more damage. We don't recommend it. Under a microscope, an aged muscle reveals a loss of cells, atrophy of cells, accumulation of fat and collagen and loss of contractility. Aging muscles are less flexible than young muscles and are more susceptible to strains, pulls and cramping. Therefore, muscle is not replaceable, so never damage it. Muscles are most efficiently trainable between the ages of 15 and 22. Train them young. Engage in only light exercise after 30.

As for the bones, there are two main types of bone problems as we age. First, the bones are worn and damaged through lifelong hard work and exercise, also known as osteoarthritis: the swelling and stiffening of the weight-bearing joints of the body. Many bone surgeries are due to damage from sports injuries acquired during youth. Second, bone problems can arise from loss of calcium and other vital essence, resulting in osteoporosis, the thinning bone condition that causes humped backs and fractures of the hip and spine.

Osteoarthritis results when the spongy cartilage, or gristle, of the joints is ground away from years of use or injury, leaving joint bones raw and unpadded. Again, exercise can be a two-edged sword. Certain forms of strenuous exercise may make us prone to osteoarthritis, particularly weight lifting, push-ups, football and baseball. Light to moderate exercise, such as jogging, biking, swimming and walking can actually help prevent arthritis by keeping the bones, ligaments and cartilage in good working order.

The back, neck, hips and knees are prone to arthritis, especially after a lifetime of sports injury, trauma or even poor posture. Ballet dancers tend to develop arthritis in their feet; tennis players tend to get it in their elbows and joggers in their knees. Obesity has been linked with arthritis, too, from joints having to bear excess weight. People who use computers all day long tend to be constantly in one posture, creating strain on the lower back.

Unlike muscles, joints register wounds at a much younger age. A twisted ankle at age 13 during a basketball game will likely be twisted in the same place many times throughout a lifetime. Even if we are young, the damage never goes away completely. It heals, but is always weaker than the original. Bone can never recover to its pre-injured strength, so it's important to avoid unnecessarily strenuous exercise.

Osteoporosis is the loss of bone density, namely thinning of the bones with reduction in bone mass due to depletion of calcium and bone protein. It predisposes a person to fractures, which are often slow to heal and heal poorly. Osteoporosis is more common in older adults, particularly in post-menopausal women and andropausal men. Unchecked osteoporosis can lead to changes in posture, physical abnormality (particularly the form of hunched back known as "dowager's hump") and decreased mobility. It can be measured using a special x-ray called a quantitative computed tomogram.

Conventional wisdom asks us to take plenty of calcium and conduct a lot of resistance training. However, hormone imbalance is the underlying cause of osteoporosis, rather than a lack of nutrients and resistance training. Young adults never have to do a lot of resistance training or take a lot of calcium in order to keep bone mass.

4.2   KEEPING YOUTHFUL FUNCTIONALITY FOR LIFE

All body mechanical functions have a range of motion from minimum to normal in a relaxed condition to maximum. When we talk about keeping functionality, we refer to keeping such range for life.

We normally lose range of motion gradually if we don't use that motion. For example, presbyopia is caused by the fiber in the lens of the eye becoming so stiff that it cannot contract enough to see near objects. This is because we normally never stretch it to its "minimum." When we get older, we lose the ability to do leg splits. This is due again to never practicing the "maximum." Many of us lose vital capacity, a measure for maximum lung function, again due to seldom practicing stretching our lung capability to the maximum. Thus if we don't often stretch our capability to its "minimum" end and "maximum" end, we gradually lose that range of functionality. We become confined! We get old!

On the other hand, from previous sections, we know that if we do too much exercise, and/or the wrong kind of exercise, we create damage to our muscles, tendons and bones, which will limit our functionality.

Therefore, Ping Longevity™ is designed to:

- Be able to reach our extreme functionality, i.e., "minimum" and "maximum" capacity very frequently, on a daily basis, if possible;

- Exercise at peak capacity for very short periods of time, seconds and minutes, to avoid overstressing the mechanical system;

- Apply functional fitness to mechanical aspects of all major body systems such as heart, lung, bones, muscles, tendons, eyes, ears and brain.

This is very different from conventional exercise, in which you're taught to exercise for a long time to potentially overstress the body creating increased wear and tear and usually focusing only in a limited way on functional areas.

4.2.1   Heart and Lung Fitness

The lungs are paired organs in the chest that perform respiration. Each human has two lungs, which are separated by a structure called the mediastinum. The mediastinum contains the heart, trachea, esophagus and blood vessels. The lungs are covered by a protective membrane called the pulmonary pleura.

Respiration is the main function of the lungs, which is the process of oxygen from incoming air entering the blood and carbon dioxide, a waste gas from the metabolism of food leaving the blood. Each day, you take about 23,000 breaths, which bring almost 10,000 quarts of air into your lungs. The air that you breathe contains several gases, including oxygen, that are essential for your cells to function. With each breath, your lungs add fresh oxygen to your blood, which then carries it to your cells.

Lung function normally peaks in the late teens and early twenties. After the early twenties, lung function declines about 1 percent a year over the rest of a person's lifetime. Lung function decreases about 2 percent a year for people who smoke.

The heart is a mechanical pump, composed of muscle that pumps blood throughout the body, beating approximately 60 to 72 times per minute for our entire lives. The heart pumps the blood, which carries all the vital materials that help our bodies function and remove waste products. For example, the brain requires oxygen and glucose, which, if not received continuously, will cause you to lose consciousness. Muscles need oxygen, glucose and amino acids, as well as the proper ratio of sodium, calcium and potassium salts in order to contract normally. The glands need sufficient supplies of raw materials from which to manufacture the specific secretions. If the heart ever ceases to pump blood, the body begins to shut down and it will die after a very short period of time.

Most of us do not often get our hearts and lungs to work to their peak maximum capacity. As a result, since we don't use the maximum capacity, we lose it gradually.

Lung capacity is measured by forced vital capacity using a spirometer, and heart capacity by a cardiac stress test using physical treadmill exercises and chemical drugs to induce stress and monitored by devices such as the EKG. As a rule of thumb, when do you achieve your near maximum capacity? It is simply when you are out of breath!

How long do you need to be out of breath? In general, Ping-Longevity™ Exercise does not want you to overuse your systems. Therefore, we want you to attain an out-of-breath condition on a daily basis, but not more than 5 to 10 minutes each time.

What exercises are the best? The ones which get you out of breath quickly and are most time efficient and convenient to you.

"I live in the big city of Tokyo. I commute everyday through the subway system, where we have to go up and down stairs a lot. I always choose not to use the escalator. Instead, I run up the stairways, so that every day, I can experience at least 3 to 5 minutes of near maximum heart rate."

—SHIGEO, TOKYO

"My house is on a hill with a 15 degree road in front. My wife and I love to walk down the road to the beach every day. When we come back up, we often run 50–100 meters up the hill. Within a matter of two minutes, we get really breathless. It really stretches our lung and heart capacity very effectively."

—ERIC, SAN CLEMENTE, CA

In the PingLongevity™ Morning Routine, as seen in Section 4.4.1, we incorporate deep squat jumps. Taoist masters often tell you that deep squats are excellent ways to stretch the most important energy center, the Hui Ying (gate of life). If you were involved in professional sports, you may remember that numerous repetitions of deep squat jumps and deep leap frog jumps are among the most dreaded exercises ordered up by the toughest coaches. If you try deep squat jumps, you'll soon know that this exercise can get you to maximum heart rate within seconds, with many other health benefits!

4.2.2   Resistance Training

Resistance training is any exercise that causes the muscles to contract against an external resistance with the expectation of increases in strength, tone, mass and/or endurance. The external resistance can be dumbbells, rubber exercise tubing, your own body weight, bricks, bottles of water or any other object that causes the muscles to contract.

The best resistance exercises are weight bearing, those that require the bones to support weight and improve bone density. Like any other body function, if we don't use our bones, we lose their density. It's been shown that resistance exercises can help preserve bone density, hence prevent osteoporosis. Usually, the wrist, hip and spine are most prone to breaking due to osteoporosis, which also causes curvature of the spine. Resistance exercises that put weights on these areas include pushups, which put resistance to wrist bones and deep squat jumps or leap frog jumps that put weight on your hip and leg bones (Section 4.4.1).

Resistance training also builds muscle strength and tone. The number of muscle fibers declines with age. From age 30 to age 70 we can lose more than 25% of the Type 2 muscle fibers in our bodies (Type 2 fibers are our strength fibers). Resistance exercise can slow down or even reverse the aging process by building muscle mass and strength.

For example, among the weakest muscle groups in most white collar office people is the so called "core muscles." Core muscles are the supporting muscles for the spine. They include the abdominal muscles, external obliques, internal obliques, rectus abdominis and the back muscle erector spinae. That's why there are so many of us with back problems. The core muscles are simply giving up on their job, leaving all the weight bearing to the spine. This frequently causes back problems, such as disc herniation.

The key is to choose a small number of highly effective exercises. Exercises that help the core muscles include horizontal leg raises, horizontal back raises, vertical leg/back raise, vertical leg side raise (Section 4.4.1).

How much do we need to do this? Remember that the goal is to retain functionality, rather than to build a significant muscle mass. Therefore, we usually recommend simply doing one set each day, so that we minimize wear and tear. How many times? You should do a number of times that is near the most you're able to do.

In resistance training, we believe it is best to use your own body weight. This makes you less prone to injury than external weights. The other advantage is that you can do these exercises anywhere.

4.2.3   Flexibility Training

Like many other range of motion exercises, reaching over to touch your toes with your knee joints straight is a functionality that you can gradually lose as you grow older. On the other hand, people who stretch their hamstrings through yoga and other exercises can keep the range for life. So it comes to the old saying, "If you don't use it, you lose it." We tend to lose flexibility with aging due to a loss in elasticity in the connective tissues surrounding the muscles that go through a normal shortening process resulting from a lack of physical activity.

Flexibility is one of the most important aspects of functional fitness because range of motion is simply the critical thing we need to live our daily lives. Flexibility refers to the total range of motion of joints. With the muscles relaxed and reflex mechanisms minimally involved, the motion of a joint is primarily determined by its joint capsule, including ligaments, muscles and their fascial sheaths, tendons.

Static, or hold stretching, is probably the most commonly used flexibility technique and is very safe and effective. With this technique, a muscle or muscle group is gradually stretched to the point of limitation and then typically held in that position for a period of 15 to 30 seconds.

The main muscle groups requiring good flexibility for most of our daily functioning are: upper body movements (neck, shoulders, triceps, torso) and lower body movements (gluts, adductor, hamstring, quadriceps, calf). If you only have time to do one stretch, then do hamstrings because that is typically the tightest muscle in the body and it can lead to back pain if it is not flexible enough.

There are many good flexibility training routines. In designing your own, you just need to make sure to cover your tightest areas. For example, you may choose the Pilates hamstring stretch for hamstrings and the deep squat jump for groin muscles. (Section 4.4.1).

4.2.4   Eye Fitness

Presbyopia is an eye condition that will generally happen to everyone. Nowadays, people get presbyopia earlier and earlier, many in their 40s. People with presbyopia have a hard time focusing up close and find themselves having to hold up reading material at arms' length to focus.

Presbyopia is caused by an age-related deterioration of the lens of the eye. This differs from astigmatism, nearsightedness and farsightedness, which are related to the shape of the eyeball and are caused by genetic and environmental factors. Presbyopia generally is believed to stem from a gradual thickening and loss of flexibility of the natural lens inside your eyes. These age-related changes occur within the proteins in the lens, making the lens harder and less elastic over time. Age-related changes also take place in the muscle fibers surrounding the lens. With less elasticity, the eye has a harder time focusing up close.

Almost none of us exercise our eyes to their "minimum" range of reading. Therefore, the lens rarely gets stretched to its limits. As a result, we gradually lose the functionality to read close up.

> "I was giving a speech to a large audience of spa owners in Beijing. At the end of the lecture, I told them that as a gift of this lecture I'd like to give them an exercise, one that will help protect their eyes against presbyopia. I told them that the reason for reading glasses is due to eye muscles losing the ability to zoom in and out. A simple yet effective exercise, while costing you no time, is the following: When you read magazines, newspapers, novels or work documents during the day, allocate three to five minutes to move the paper as far from your eyes as you can still read for one paragraph, then move it as close as you can to your eyes for another paragraph. Alternate between far and near positions from paragraph to paragraph.'"
>
> —DR. TAICHI TZU

4.2.5 Hearing Protection

We actually don't want to exercise our hearing to the maximum if we can avoid it. That's because ears are like drums. Every day when we hear things, we beat that drum. If the sound is too loud, the drum is beaten harder, thus it wears out faster. You often see older people cupping their hands behind an ear to try to hear what you are saying. That's because they have lost their hearing through wear and tear.

To stay young, we'd like to protect our eardrums! The best friend to our eardrums is a pair of high rated ear plugs. Ear plugs are rated through noise reduction rating (NRR). You need to use an ear plug with NRR higher than 30 db.

You need to use ear plugs for dance clubs and bars where loud music is played, for riding airplanes (noise and pressure), if you're riding a motorcycle or operating a lawn mower or any occasions where there is a high noise level.

4.2.6   Brain Fitness

"I have started to forget things. I'm groping for words and sometimes I have to really concentrate to find my way home from an unfamiliar place. I am really worried. I don't want to get Alzheimer's."

We often hear something like this from our older friends and relatives. Alzheimer's is the most dreaded disease! However, signs of Alzheimer's are very commonplace to many people, as published by the American Alzheimer's Association:

- Memory changes that disrupt daily life;

- Challenges in planning or solving problems;

- Difficulty completing familiar tasks at home, at work, or at leisure;

- Confusion with time or place;

- Trouble understanding visual images and spatial relationship;

- Trouble following or joining a conversation;

- Misplacing things and losing the ability to retrace steps;

- Decreased or poor judgment;

- Withdrawal from work or social activities;

- Change in mood and personality.

Early signs of brain functional decline can also be accurately tested through a process called the brain electrical activity map (BEAM). That's why we recommend an annual BEAM test as part of the PingLongevity™ Test (Section 1.4.4) protocols.

The human brain is able to continually adapt and rewire itself.

Even in old age, it can grow new neurons. Severe mental decline is usually caused by disease, whereas most age-related losses in memory or motor skills simply result from inactivity and a lack of mental exercise and stimulation. In other words again, use it or lose it.

Two areas of the brain are more prone to damage and deterioration over time. One is the hippocampus, which transfers new memories to long-term storage elsewhere in the brain. Another vulnerable area is the basal ganglia, which coordinates commands to move muscles. This is why remote memories aren't usually affected by aging. But your recent memory may be affected. For example, you may forget names of people you've met today or where you set your keys. You also lose coordination. Simply try to stand on one leg, with eyes closed. You start to lose the ability to balance for a few seconds.

Contrary to popular myth, you do not lose mass quantities of brain cells as you get older. Dr. Monte S. Buchsbaum, director of the Neuroscience PET Laboratory at Mount Sinai School of Medicine conducted an experiment, in which 6000 people were given mental tests throughout a 10-year period. Almost 70% continued to maintain their brainpower throughout the period.

"There isn't much difference between a 25-year-old brain and a 75-year-old brain."
—Dr. Monte Buchsbaum

Cognitive decline is not inevitable. Research indicates that mental exercise can improve these areas and positively affect memory and physical coordination.

A Case Western Reserve University Medical School study of 550 people, led by Dr. Amir Soas found those less mentally and physically active in middle age were three times more likely to get Alzheimer's as they grayed.

Besides being intellectually active, there many specialized brain activities can exercise the brain.

For example, the following exercises are highly effective, yet require very little dedicated time:

- Static balance chi-gong is a very good exercise. You can do this anywhere, for example, while you're standing in line waiting for a cashier (Section.4.4.1).

- Do routine tasks, such as getting dressed for work, taking a shower, performing yoga with your eyes closed;

- Eat a meal with your family in silence using only visual cues;

- Listen to a specific piece of music while smelling a particular aroma.

- Use your opposite hand to brush your teeth, dial the phone or operate the TV remote.

These are exercises designed to help your brain manufacture its own nutrients that strengthen, preserve and grow brain cells and activate underused nerve pathways and connections, helping you achieve a fit and flexible mind. They can be done anywhere, anytime, in offbeat, fun and easy ways.

4.3   NEGATIVE-G THERAPY

In this section, we discuss an anti-aging therapy called negative-G therapy. It utilizes negative gravity to achieve many health benefits.

4.3.1   Body under Gravity

What is gravity, or g-force? Galileo was probably the first to look closely at the way objects fall to Earth. Legend has it that he climbed to the top of the leaning tower of Pisa and from there simultaneously dropped heavy and light balls, noting that they hit the ground at the same time. He thus demonstrated, contrary to some ancient claims, that heavy and light objects fell at the same rate.

A dropped object starts its fall quite slowly, but then steadily increases velocity. The velocity of a ball dropped from a high place increases each second by a constant amount, usually denoted by the small letter "g" (for gravity). The number for g, usually called the acceleration factor of gravity, is approximately 9.8. Thus, influenced by gravity, an object drops at a speed which increases by 9.8 meters (32 feet) per second.

Following Galileo, Isaac Newton continued the study of force. Among his many great discoveries, Newton learned the relationship among the force (F) that acts on an object, the mass (M) of the object and its acceleration factor (a) (in the case of gravity, a is the same as g). In his celebrated first law of motion, the relationship is described by the following formula: $F = Ma$, or $F = Mg$ in the case of gravity.

Gravity, or g-force, is the large force acting upon us, which equals our weight. Think about this force pulling down the heart, liver, stomach, blood in the vessels, lymph fluids, etc. Luckily, we have all kinds of tissues pulling our organs up in place and our heart pumping blood upward to supply the brain and the upper extremities. However, for a 50-year-old person, he or she has been under this force for 50 years, constantly. When we stand straight up, all of our vertical structures are especially affected by such a force. Our spines are compressed as we move under such force. No wonder we become shorter as we age: All of our bones are compressed at the discs and joints. Our organs, too, are pulled down as we age. The lower abdomen becomes larger, even without added fat.

We often hear about people having lowered stomachs. This is because the mechanisms for holding the organs in place (muscles, tendons, ligaments and other membranes) are pulled and stretched over many years. Gravity pulls body fat downward as we age. We grow eye bags and double chins as the fat is pulled downward. More fat is pulled to the belly, hips and thighs. Gravity also makes the buttocks and breasts sag. When we notice that everything is a half an inch lower, we feel the impact of aging. Furthermore, the blood is affected by gravity, too. When your heart is strong, this is okay. However, as the heart weakens with age, its ability to counter gravity by pumping blood up to the head and other small vessels in the upper parts of the body is diminished. Thus, the heart is more stressed and the head is less nourished by blood. Gravity also increases metabolic rates, since the body has to counter the g-force.

Can we do away with gravity? No. We cannot live without gravity. Each part of us, through billions of years of evolution since our non-human ancestors climbed out of the ocean, has adapted to gravity. During short gravity-free periods, we can temporarily lose our ability to fight gravity. A person on bed rest for too long can easily faint when he stands up because he loses his ability to withstand the g-force.

Man co-exists with gravity; without it, we simply cannot live. But gravity is also part of nature's way that wears us down. Do we accept it or can we do something to lessen the negative impact?

Our circulatory systems have adapted to vertical gravity. We are able to maintain an adequate supply of blood to the brain in the upright posture despite the heart having to pump the blood upward against gravity. This is made possible by certain compensatory mechanisms, which cause the small blood vessels in the legs to constrict, thus preventing the blood from pooling down. Our sensory mechanisms are in the right heart ventricle. If the blood volume is low due to blood pulled down by g-force, several hormones, including rennin, aldosterone and catecholamines, kick into action to stimulate a contraction of peripheral blood vessels, such as the ones in the legs. The contraction creates a narrower path for the blood downward and higher resistance (or blood pressure), thus making more blood available for the head.

Staying only a few days in a weightless environment or simply on bed rest, results in biological deterioration. This is called a sub-g environment. Under such conditions, the vascular systems in the lower extremities do not need to restrict blood since there is no downward pulling by the g-force. After a while, you temporarily lose the capability. A sudden return to normal gravity—such as a space shuttle reentry, or sitting up after a long-term bed rest—may cause fainting because blood cannot be effectively restricted from pouring downwards. The brain does not have a sufficient supply of oxygen and glucose carried by blood. On the other hand, life in a hyper-gravity environment, such as may be experienced on a planet with 1.5 times the earth's gravity, would be miserable; we would have to lie down all the time due to an insufficient supply of blood to the head if we straightened up. It would also increase the evolutionary rate of development of bipedalism so that our lower blood vessels can restrict more.

The sub-g and hyper-g situation can be easily felt on an airplane ride. Remember your last flight? At takeoff, as the plane ascends, we experience a force more than the normal g, a hyper-g situation, because we are traveling opposite of the g-force. We are adapted to the normal g. When we are experiencing higher g force, our usual blood restriction mechanism is not sufficient. Therefore, we feel a temporary shortage of oxygen supply to the head: a faint feeling. To combat the additional g-force, the heart has to pump more blood to sustain the requirements of the brain. This in turn requires a higher metabolic rate and higher energy consumption. We can also feel the higher g-force drag our organs down lower than normal. Our muscles and ligaments are stretched further in order to hold the organs in place. These are some reasons that we tire easily after a flight.

As our plane descends, we experience a g-force that is a fraction of the usual because we are dropping in the same direction as gravity is pulling. The head is now flushed with blood and the organs are suspended upward. To respond to this, the heart slows down and pumps less blood to the head. The metabolic rate slows down too.

Flight just amplifies the sensation that something abnormal has happened to our physiology and autonomous control systems. On the ground, we are so used to the normal g-force that we don't even think of it. We forget about the force exerted on us every minute, every day of our lives.

Much of life is about fighting gravity. Why does the heart pump harder when we run than when we sit still? It is because we fight harder against gravity.

Dr. Esar Shvartz presented a series of scientific experiments in his book *Biogravics*. It was shown that immersion in water produced a heart rate of 50, as compared to 60 for a recumbent position, 70 for a sitting position, 80 for standing, 110 for walking, and 140 for running. As gravity increases, the heart has to pump harder to supply blood to the upper extremities. Being immersed in water is the easiest. We do not need to fight against gravity, largely because water provides the counteractive force to balance the gravitational pull. It usually makes us very relaxed.

Sitting, standing and walking represent three other states. In a recumbent position, no attempt is made to oppose gravity except for the semiconscious metabolic functions. In sitting, an attempt is made to emerge from this condition. Man can maintain a sitting position for several hours, even though it requires substantial adjustments with respect to weight distribution, balance and blood pooling. Some people with low blood pressure have difficulty sitting upright for prolonged periods because they experience dizzy spells due to insufficient blood pressure in the brain. When a quick change is made from a recumbent to a sitting position, momentary dizziness may be experienced because of a delay in the compensatory increase in arterial blood pressure, which occurs to provide an adequate supply of blood to the brain.

Standing is an important human evolutionary capacity, which has not yet reached perfection. Up to 20% of healthy young men faint when standing motionless for only twenty minutes because of blood pooling in the legs and abdomen (pulled down by gravity) and lack of blood supply to the brain. In most cases, this happens when they are consciously trying to avoid movement, such as when standing at military attention, an unnatural posture. Most people do not faint when standing in a relaxed position because the leg muscle action helps to pump the blood up against gravity. However, even relaxed standing cannot be tolerated by humans for prolonged periods.

4.3.2   The Negative-G Condition

What if we are under reverse gravity positions, i.e., a negative-g environment? This is when the head is lower than the feet in an inversely tilted position or completely upside down position. We may all have experienced this in our lives. Untrained people cannot be upside down for long. It's unbearable. What about a tilted position? Depending on the degree of tilt, we may tolerate it for shorter or longer periods.

Despite our general intolerance for a negative-g situation, we may gain some benefit from it. From a common-sense point of view, we would guess that the heart rate would slow, the metabolic rate decrease, the downward pulling of organs, fat, skin, etc., would be reversed. There is a potential added benefit too. In fact, as we get older, our ability to fight against g-force diminishes. An older person suddenly moving from a head-down to a head-up position easily gets dizzy because blood cannot be sufficiently supplied to the head. An older person also has difficulty supplying enough blood to the head, causing deteriorating brain function. Similar to exercising muscles, a negative-g force may train our brains, hormones and peripheral vascular systems to respond to g-force effectively even as we age. Thus, a negative-g force may enable us to live longer and look younger.

Winged birds typically outlive comparable sized land mammals. Bats outlive rats by a factor of six to four. Of the 4000-odd species of mammals on the earth, nearly one-quarter of them are bats. Are they a strong species because they live mostly horizontal or inverted? Or because they do not need to fight gravity as hard as the same size land mammal? Is it because bats sleep head down? Why are most ocean mammals ageless? Is it partially due to their near-zero gravity environment?

There have been many studies about the negative-g conditions in the area of aerospace medicine in the '50s and '60s due to the advancement of the space program and the international space station. The studies provide us much data on the hypothesis of the impact of negative-g on longevity.

Dr. Lawrence Lamb and Captain James Roman, USAF, performed a pioneering study published in the June 1961 volume of *Aerospace Medicine* on the circulatory response from +1g (in a normal standing position) to 0g (recumbent bed rest or weightlessness), and −1g force (in an upside-down position). A total of 224 subjects participated in the study. Under +1g, the sympathetic control of the circulatory system is stimulated. Through sympathetic influences, peripheral veins are contracted to restrict blood from pouring downward. Thus, peripheral resistance is maintained, which in turn provides for adequate distribution of cardiac output. This also increases heartbeat and blood pressure. When a sympathetic stimulation is dominant, it is common to see cardiac acceleration or an increased heart rate. In a recumbent position or bed rest, a transverse +1g force is acting on us, so it is a close approximation of a weightless situation for the circulatory system from head to feet. This will result in a cardiac system slowdown with slower heartbeat and relaxation of peripheral vascular resistance. In a head-down tilt situation simulating a negative-g, the heartbeat and peripheral vascular resistance are even more relaxed.

A study of hormonal response to a 10-degree head-down tilt (negative g-force) as compared to a standing position was conducted by Dr. Claude Gharib and others, published in the July 1988 and January 1992 issues of *Aerospace Medicine*. Under such a negative-g force, the contractility of the right ventricle (measured by the mean rate of right ventricular pressure) decreased by 34%, and the work performed reduced by 27%. There is a 15% progressive increase in plasma volume (more blood available) and an 18% decrease in diastolic blood pressure. There are also hormonal changes: plasma renin activity reduced by 60%, aldosterone by 63%, and catecholamines by 20%.

In summary, under a negative-g condition, metabolic rate and the downward compression of organs, skin and spine are dramatically decreased. The head is supplied with ample blood to nourish its functioning. There is a strong hypothesis that a scientific negative-g therapy is critical to longevity.

4.3.3   Method to Achieving Negative-G

The scientific rationale for using negative-g on longevity was first proposed by Dr. Taichi Tzu in 2003.

Before presenting the method, we must stress again that all negative-g methods are based on empirical experience, as well as aerospace research oriented to the study of space shuttle physiology rather than longevity. Our readers are advised to consult with certified physicians before practicing the negative-g therapy.

There are several ways of practicing zero to negative g. For example, water sports. Since immersing in water provides a nice near zero g environment, most water sports are good for health, such as swimming and water aerobics. Being in water is less stressful than equivalent land positions. Another example is upside-down exercise. An ancient Chinese chi-gong practice by the monks starts with a long period of standing upside down, using the hands as support. Gradually, one moves to a one-handed support and finally to one finger supporting the whole body. It was believed that this practice increases longevity. There are many other ways of being upside down, such as certain yoga postures, gymnastics exercises and using tilt tables.

However, all these methods are limited because the time spent in daily or weekly exercises in a negative-g environment is very negligible as compared to a whole life span under the constant pull of positive-g. In order to create a real impact, negative-g has to be a significant part of our life, rather than a one-hour per week exercise.

PingLongevity™ Negative-g Therapy: The idea is strikingly simple and the effect is dramatic. If we are able to sleep every night head down on bed tiled 10 to 20 degrees, assuming eight-hours of sleep per day, we would have an equivalent 6 to 10% of our lifetime in a full negative 1g environment. To be clear, for each 24-hour day, we would be spending an equivalent of 2.4 hours in a straight head-down feet-up position. Note that this therapy uses a straight tilted bed rather than beds that bend at the middle.

By using PingLongevity™ Negative-g Therapy, we can achieve 6 to 10% of a lifetime in a full negative 1g environment to counter the daily downward pull on organs, skin and blood. In such a negative-g environment, we that bend at the middle. practice increases longevity. The heart simply does not work as hard. Our real-life five-year experience confirms this. It has been a lot easier to get into very deep sleep and rest.

In summary, negative-g therapy can be a significant part of life rather than an exercise with negligible duration. PingLongevity™ Negative-g Therapy is a break-

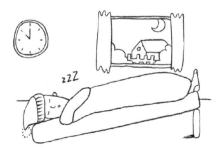

through method to achieve 6–10% of full negative 1g environment during the entire lifetime. Be sure to consult with certified physicians before trying this method because of its limited scientific data in the area of anti-aging and risk evaluation.

4.4   IMPLEMENTATION OF FUNCTIONAL FITNESS

Chapter 4 has given you an overview of the methodology of Ping-Longevity™ Exercise. In this section, we give you a simple set of exercises.

Most of us don't have time to do a lot of exercise. In fact, from functional fitness point of view, devoting a large chunk of time is neither necessary nor desirable. The following is a 10- to 20-minute daily 11-exercise routine, which will get you to optimal functionality.

PingLongevity™ Morning Routine:

1. **Vertical Leg Back Raise:** Stand straight facing a wall, as closely as possible, with your hands slightly supported by the wall. Tighten your stomach muscle. Slowly raise one leg backwards as high as you can, while keeping the entire body parallel to the wall, knees straight. Slowly drop the leg down without touching the floor. Repeat 20 times. Repeat on the other side.

2. **Vertical Leg Side Raise:** Stand straight facing a wall as closely as possible, with your hands lightly supported by the wall. Tighten your stomach muscles. Slowly raise one leg sideways as high as you can, while keeping the entire body parallel to the wall, knees straight. Slowly drop the leg down without touching the floor. Repeat 20 times. Repeat on the other side.

3. **Narrow Pushup:** The only difference here from regular pushup is that when you push up, you must keep your elbows at the same width as your shoulders, your hands pointing forward and your body in a straight line. In the lowered position, you must be low enough so that your elbows bend less than 90 degrees. Repeat 20 or as many repetitions as you can under these parameters.

4. **Horizontal Leg Raise:** Lie face up on the floor, hands behind your head. Slowly raise both legs to near vertical, while keeping knees straight. Lower the legs without touching the floor. Do not raise your head from the floor. Your head and upper body must remain on the floor all the time. Repeat 20 times, or as much as you can in the proper position.

5. **Pilates Hamstring Stretch:** Lie face up on the floor. With a towel or a rope wrapped around one foot, pull on the rope to raise the leg as much as possible while keeping the knee straight and the rest of the body still. Hold for 10 to 20 seconds, pull a little more on the rope or towel and hold for another 10 to 20 seconds, then pull even more for another 10 to 20 seconds. Repeat 20 times, and repeat on the other side.

6. **Cross Leg Knee Hug:** Lie face up on the floor. With both legs straight, cross one leg on top of the other, ankle over knee. Bend the straight leg underneath to 90 degree angle with the foot flat on the floor. Use both hands to pull the knee of the non-crossed leg towards your chest. Hold for 10 to 20 seconds, pull in more, hold for another 10–20 seconds, then pull even more for another 10 to 20 seconds. Repeat 20 times, then repeat on the other side.

7. **Closed-Eye Handstand:** Stand on both hands, arms straight, with your entire body vertically inverted against a wall. Close your eyes. Vertically stand for as long as you can. NOTE: It's a good idea to have a helper with you for the first few times to be sure you don't topple over.

8. **Deep Squat Jump:** Deep squat as low as you can. Then jump up as high as you can. Repeat 20 times, or as many as you can.

9. **Straight Crawl Forward/Backward:** Starting from a position with you hands and feet on the floors arms and knees straight, hands and feet about 1 $1/2$ times shoulder width apart. Keeping your spine and upper body straight, crawl forward with first the right knee moving to touch the right elbow, then the left knee touching the left elbow. Move about 20 steps in this

manner, depending on the size of the room. Then backward with reversing the same movement. Do this for two repetitions.

10. **Static Balance Chi-Gong:** Stand on a hard surface (not on a rug), close your eyes, and get into chi-gong state. Calm your mind, modulate your breath (Section 6.4.1). Then, lift one foot about 6 inches off the ground, bending your free knee at about a 45-degree angle. Remain still for as long as you can. Repeat on the other side.

11. **PingLongevity™ Anti-Presbyopia Exercise:** Spend 3–5 minutes reading magazines, newspapers, novels or work documents. Move the paper as far from your eyes as you can still read for one paragraph, then move it as close as you can to your eyes for another paragraph. Alternate between far and near positions from paragraph to paragraph.

4.5   SUMMARY

PingLongevity™ Exercise focuses on keeping the body's functionality, at youthful levels for life. It is not designed to burn fat or to achieve a gold medal in sports, or even for recreational fun. It utilizes exercises that are either part of a daily task or consume very little time. The following is a summary:

• Your exercise routine must exercise the heart and lungs, put resistance on the bones, stretch the ranges of joints, muscles and tendons, exercise the eyes, protect hearing, stimulate the brain and brain-body connections;

• Your job is to do as little exercise as possible, so as not to create wear and tear, in order to retain the maximum range of functionality in each of the body systems;

• Utilize exercises built into your daily routine, or consuming very little time so as to be able to persist for a long period of time;

• Adapt the PingLongevity™ Morning Routine as a sample exercise regime. Whenever appropriate, substitute any segment with one that most fits your own body's needs.

CHAPTER 5

Balance Energy Meridians

In this chapter, we'll discuss PingLongevity™ Energy Balance. Traditional Chinese Medicine believes that the imbalance of energy meridians is a fundamental cause of disease. That's the principle of acupuncture. It is also the principle of many chi-gong methods that focus on specific energy centers.

Balancing your body's energy system is an integral part of Ping - Longevity™. It is drastically different from conventional medicine's method of treating one or a small number of symptoms at one time. We often see patients taking too many drugs, yet doctors can't resist prescribing even more for them. Patients may start with anti-inflammatory drugs for joint and muscle pain, but soon their stomachs hurt due to the side effects. So the doctor has to put them on a stomach pill. Often they become depressed from the pain. So they have to take an antidepressant drug or mood medicine. Their sleep is disturbed and they use sleeping pills. Some of these patients take medication ten times a day. It's a vicious cycle. They must take medicine. It is prescribed. Then come the side effects and they take more drugs.

Indeed, according to a new statistics cited by *USA Today*, more than 44% of Americans take prescription drugs daily. Approximately 9% take more than five prescription drugs a day.

A similar phenomenon happens in nutritional medicine. You may take vitamins A, B, C, D, E and lots more. New nutrients and supplements that the body requires are discovered every day, nutrients that are good for diabetes, joints, heart, lung, pain, etc. You don't want to miss any, so you take more. Every single one of these nutrients and supplements is good for some part of the body. So pretty soon, you take 30 to 50 capsules a day.

All of us have three major planes of being: the physical plane, the energy plane and the spiritual plane. They range from lower to higher energy frequencies of the universe as will be discussed in Chapter 10.

Until now, when we have discussed diet, exercise and caloric restriction, we were talking about the physical plane. This chapter will devoted to the energy plane. We will talk about how to get chi balanced and flowing unobstructed through the body meridians (energy channels). We will introduce methods that focus on the major energy meridians. Once they are balanced, many symptoms and diseases go away. Best of all, you may be able use the methods as a self healing tool without doctors. The method is simple, but powerful.

> "James was treated for low back pain. After a few weeks of taking kidney support herbs, his pain was completely eased. In his last visit, he asked what I did to him, as for now his tinnitus (ringing in the ears), a problem he never told me he had experienced for years, had disappeared as well. I had been trying to strengthen his internal kidney meridians. When the kidneys are strong, all kidney-related symptoms go away. Ear ringing and low back pain are both related to kidney energy. So taking the kidney support herbs balanced the energy. This is why both symptoms are gone, even though we did not specifically treat the tinnitus."
>
> —DR. PING

Like blood, chi (energy) is the sustaining force of every part of us. It flows invisibly through energy channels, called meridians in Traditional Chinese Medicine (TCM). These meridians are not physically seen and don't correspond to anything in anatomy. However, plenty of modern scientific research has proven that such higher subtle energy exists. Chi can be partially measured and has some property of electromagnetic energy. Meridians are also proven to be along low electrical resistant points in the body, the so-called acupuncture points.

Once the energy is balanced and vibrant, the body is free from all diseases and in a state of maximum vitality. This is exactly the principle of acupuncture and herbal medicine. When energy is blocked, or unbalanced, it flows through the meridians in an unbalanced way. Acupuncture needles inserted at energy points along meridians cause the meridian to rebalance its stagnated energy flow due to the stimulation and sometimes the energy transmission from the acupuncturist's hands. We use acupuncture when we are sick. In order to have vibrant health, we want to open and balance our meridians automatically every minute throughout the whole body, ideally before we get sick.

There are many reasons meridians get blocked and unbalanced. The environment puts us through many emergency responses that necessarily pull us off balance. When we face a stressful situation, our systems automatically release hormones to instruct the body to shut down normal body processes, such as digestion, and focus all energy on the emergency at hand. You can instantly feel your heart pump faster. When you catch a cold, your body has to declare a state of emergency (high fever, for instance) to deal with the situation. When our normal perfect equilibrium is off balance, we don't return exactly to the same place after the crisis has passed. In fact, the post-stress state is usually far from equilibrium. We settle down at a new unbalanced energy place. Thus the body starts to work sub-optimally. The situation is made worse by modern materialism: increased cravings for money, fame and power, more than formerly accepted standards, thus becoming contrary to our original nature. We turn natural desires, for example the desire for sex, into indulgence. We become the hardest working species on earth. As a result, there is a heightened trend toward unbalanced energy meridians.

The Yellow Emperor's Classic of Medicine is the most authoritative book on TCM, written by the great Huang Di, the Yellow Emperor, who reigned in China 5,000 years ago. In it, there is the following dialog between Huang Di and his advisor Qi Bo:

Huang Di asked, "I have heard that in ancient times, when the sages treated, all they had to do was employ methods to guide and change the emotional and spiritual state of a person and redirect the energy flow. The sages utilized a method called zhu you: prayer, ceremony and shamanism that healed all conditions. Today, however, when doctors treat a patient, they use herbs to treat the internal aspect and acupuncture to treat the external. Yet some conditions do not respond to this treatment. Why is this?"

Qi Bo answered, "In ancient times, people lived simply. They hunted, fished and were with nature all day. When the weather cooled, they became active to fend off the cold. When the weather heated up in summer, they retreated to cool places. Internally, their emotions were calm and peaceful and they were without excessive desires. Externally, they did not have the stresses that most of us experience today. They lived without greed and desire, close to nature. They maintained jing shen nei suo, or inner peace and concentration of the mind and spirit. This prevented pathogens from invading their systems and contributing to illness. Therefore, they did not need herbs to treat their internal state, nor did they need acupuncture to treat the external. When they did contract disease, they simply guided properly the emotions and spirit and redirected the energy flow, using the method of zhu you to heal the condition.

"People today are different. Internally, they are enslaved by their emotions and worries. They work too hard in heavy labor. They do not follow the rhythmic changes of the four seasons and thus become susceptible to the invasion of the thieves or winds. When their zheng, anti-pathogenic chi, is weak, pathogens invade to destroy the five zang organs, the bone, and the marrow. Externally, they are attacked via the sensory orifices, the skin and muscles. Thus mild conditions become severe and severe conditions turn fatal. At this point, the method of zhu you would be insufficient."

—*THE YELLOW EMPEROR'S CLASSIC OF MEDICINE*

There are two main methods of balancing our energy systems besides acupuncture, far infrared, homeopathy and magnetic therapy: (1) the herbal method, which uses a system of herbs to balance the body's energy meridians and (2) chi-gong. *Chi* or as it is sometimes spelled, *Qi* in Chinese means "of energy" and *gong* means "work." So chi-gong is the work to balance and direct the flow of chi through the meridians.

5.1   YIN AND YANG AND THE FIVE ELEMENTS

Chinese medicine has the longest undisturbed history of compiling knowledge, from the shamans of ancient folklore to modern-day physicians and scientists, spanning 5,000 years of wisdom that integrates the art with the science of healing.

> "Is holistic medicine a science? The mainstream belief is that alternative medicine therapies such as Traditional Chinese Medicine, most of them thousands of years old, are not based on science, rather they are based on trial and error without rigorous scientific experiments to verify their validity.
>
> When I was at Harvard studying statistics and stochastic processes, we were taught that you can derive to an accurate statistical average, either through averaging over many short samples, such as the method used in most scientific studies, or through observation, or by averaging over a single sample path for a long time. Both may converge to the same statistical mean under the correct conditions!
>
> This shows that many holistic medicine modalities, based on thousands of years of trial and error, are in fact, also scientifically based."
>
> —DR. TAICHI TZU

Every disease is the result of an imbalance of the yin and yang of meridians and major organs. There are more than 3,000 Chinese herbs and thousands of combination formulas developed in the 5,000 years of Chinese medicine. These are time-proven formulas noted in classic TCM. However, application of these formulas is complex. Each formula is used to compensate or cool down a particular symptom of disease. It becomes more of an art than a repeatable science.

Traditional Chinese doctors, the artists, use their own combinations of herbs and their own method of acupuncture to treat patients. Many of the formulas are passed down from generation to generation. Only male members of the family have the privilege of inheriting the secret methods. Likewise, acupuncture can be applied to many points and combinations of points, depending on the acupuncturist. The effectiveness of acupuncture is also dependent on the chi (energy) through the hands of the healers. That explains why the variation of effectiveness of herbal formulas and acupuncture treatment is so large among individual acupuncturists, like the artist who creates an oil painting: Certain artists can make a tremendous impact on the art form.

Western medicine is different. Based on symptoms, doctors order a battery of tests (blood work, x-rays, CT, urine tests and more) to diagnose patients. Once positive results are achieved, a prescribed set of medical protocols (not invented by the doctors, but provided by a few large pharmaceutical companies and approved by the government regulatory agencies) is administrated (drugs, chemotherapy). Western medicine is theoretically science-based. It certainly is not an art form.

Combining the best of TCM with the Western variety, to make this available to all people and to reduce the variations of quality provided by practitioners is the goal for all of us who are seeking good health. This not only requires standardization in formulas but also simplicity in application, which is admittedly one of the hurdles that prevents TCM from maximum availability and effectiveness for all.

In order to develop a much more simplified herbal protocol for health and longevity, let's first discuss some very basic concepts in TCM.

5.1.1 Yin-Yang Principle

Yin and yang are two opposite poles. Without yin, there is no yang. They must co-exist to make a whole. Examples are cold and hot, low and high, wet and dry, earth and heaven, north and south. When yin and yang are not equal, the equilibrium is broken.

In human health, yin mostly refers to essence or substance: blood, semen, hormones, saliva, enzymes, etc. Yang refers to energy (chi) to sustain the body's activities. For example, the heart is yang in transferring blood and the blood is yin. The heart energy to transport blood and the availability of blood form the yin and yang aspects of the heart meridian system. If the heart energy is low, the transportation of blood lacks vitality. If blood is lacking, the body cannot be nourished. To treat heart meridian-related diseases, we must first identify whether a yang deficiency or a yin deficiency is the underlying cause. Then we use herbs that can treat the corresponding deficiency to heal the body.

In general, there are four types of yin and yang imbalance:

• too strong yin, which impairs yang

• too strong yang, which over consumes yin

• deficiency in yin;

• deficiency in yang.

In the ancient classic *Plain Questions,* it was said that "a deficiency of yang brings on exterior cold, while a deficiency of yin leads to interior heat. A preponderance of yang leads to exterior heat, while a preponderance of yin leads to interior cold." Using the heart example, when yang is deficient (e.g., lack of heart energy), the symptom is a pale face, a thin, white-coated tongue, depression, etc. This is because the circulation of blood is not strong.

5.1.2 The Five Elements

The concept of the five-element theory was developed several thousand years ago. The ancient Chinese came up with the system to describe the relationships and changes in nature. They used five phenomena of earth and heaven to symbolize and provide analogies for all things in the universe. The medical application of the five-element theory is only one of its many uses.

These five phenomena are earth, water, metal, wood, and fire.

The relationship is that earth promotes metal (think about gold formed in the earth), metal promotes water, water promotes wood, wood promotes fire and fire promotes earth (by burning down things to return to the earth). You can see the cycle that makes nature a self-sustaining loop. The five elements also overcome each other. Water overcomes fire, fire overcomes metal, metal overcomes wood, wood overcomes earth (when roots cut into earth) and earth overcomes water (by blocking water). The relationship is illustrated at right.

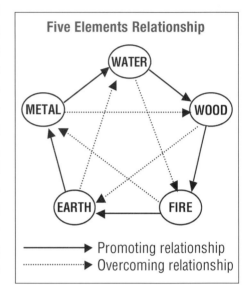

We can apply the five-element theory to many natural phenomena. Its application provides another cornerstone besides yin-yang in TCM. The human body is classified by five large energy meridian systems: the heart, lung, spleen, liver and kidney. These are not mere organs in the conventional medical sense but are systems that function as organs as well as energy systems.

For example, from a mechanical view of modern medicine, the spleen is considered part of the lymphatic system. The spleen filters blood and produces antibodies—the white blood cells. It is also considered somewhat noncritical. Often you hear about surgical removal of a spleen due to liver disease or injury in an auto accident. Nevertheless, the spleen system is considered extremely important in TCM. The spleen system connects to the stomach, governing transportation and transformation of food and dominates muscles and limbs. An impaired spleen function results in mental turmoil, often marked by irritability, poor memory and flaccid limbs. It manifests itself in the mouth (appetite, taste) and lips (pale, swollen).

These five main energy systems are put in the language of five elements in order to study the interrelationship: fire is associated with heart, earth with spleen, kidney with water, lung with metal and liver with wood. These are not random associations but are based on the interrelationship of these meridian systems. It is a demonstration that TCM thinks of the human body as a whole. When a lung is in trouble, unlike conventional medicine that treats the lung (metal), TCM looks also into spleen because spleen is earth, which promotes metal. It also looks into the heart (fire) because fire overcomes metal. Too strong a heart energy or too weak a spleen function will weaken lung energy. When the body is considered interrelated in the energy sense, rather than Western medicine's view of the body as a network of mechanical parts, it becomes very complex.

Another example of the difference between TCM and modern medicine is shown in the treatment of osteoporosis, a disease in which calcium is lost from the bones, resulting in reduced bone density. Modern medicine recommends dietary supplements of vitamin D and calcium in the hope the bones will absorb more nutrients. Recent scientific progress also makes bone replacement possible. On the other hand, traditional Chinese medicine considers bone problems a kidney deficiency.

In TCM, kidney systems not only filter blood, get rid of waste and toxins and reabsorb nutrients and minerals, including calcium and magnesium, but also represent the sex hormonal systems. If the kidney system is healthy and enough calcium and magnesium are in the diet, kidneys can reabsorb sufficient calcium and magnesium into the body. Vitamin D is also converted to its active form of D3 in the kidney system. With sufficient stores of vitamin D, calcium and magnesium can be absorbed into the bones. Thus, your body can restore your bone health through strengthening your kidney function. Since we are not growing taller, our requirement for large doses of calcium is not very high. In general, it is not that we don't have enough calcium in our diets, it is our weakened kidney function after middle age that causes problems. Thus we must treat the root cause of the bone disease and consider the body as a whole system instead of an assembly of mechanical parts. Recently, scientific studies have confirmed that a sex hormone deficiency or imbalance can result in loss of bone density, agreeing with TCM, as will be discussed in Chapter 7.

5.2   HERBAL METHODS OF ENERGY BALANCING

Symptoms are often early signs of systemic imbalance. Symptoms are the daily reports the body gives us through our senses and observations. Diseases in their infancy may or may not develop into severe illness. Most of the time, the early symptoms are not associated with the definition of disease in the context of modern medicine. Frequently, we go to a doctor telling him about our pain or inability to sleep well. The doctor tells us that nothing is wrong or that he can do nothing. This is because the symptoms have not yet developed into medically defined "diseases."

However, in the sense of preventive medicine, we know there must be some small imbalance happening. We must correct it. If not, the small imbalances will mushroom into larger ones. If we don't take the reports from our bodies' inborn messengers, we will later find out that the invaders have become too strong for us to throw out. We must deal with these early symptoms ourselves. We need to inspect ourselves every day.

5.2.1   TCM Observation Methods

TCM uses several diagnostic methods: look (e.g., face, hands, nails), listen (e.g., voice, breathing), ask questions, feel the pulse, check body temperature, smell (e.g., body odor), palpate (e.g., abdominal, lymph). Even with today's modern medicine, these methods are still important. How we feel and look is more important than simply what test results show. Many times, people who have reported symptoms to doctors and gone through batteries of tests that showed only negative results finally wound up seeing a psychologist, thinking maybe their problem was mental rather than physical. We have seen so many patients who have symptoms such as pain, but tests show nothing abnormal. But this pain is accompanied by symptoms that do mean something in the Chinese medicine method, such as red, irritated eyes or a red or pale coating on the tongue or a weak or thin, tight pulse. The pain is due to meridian blockage and organ imbalance and is not serious enough for scientific tests to show abnormal results. But if left untreated, these imbalances will develop into serious disease.

Let's talk in more detail about observation. A person's face is a very good place to read internal conditions. A pale face indicates anemia or heart energy deficiency. A rusty, dark face color could be kidney energy imbalance. Bags or dark circles under and around the eyes may come from liver imbalance. Acne, pimples, or rashes may be the sign of lung disease. Yellow color may be due to liver or spleen imbalance. A blue purplish face or lips may be the stagnation of heart blood.

Eyes are very important too. They are associated with the liver. Red swelling, pressure in the eyes or yellow sclera suggests the liver is congested, chi blocked, associated with high blood pressure, bad temper and insomnia.

Nasal discharge, running nose and a red nose all suggest lung imbalance. Ear is associated with kidney. Dry withered auricles or a burnt black color suggest the kidney is under stress. Gum redness and swelling could be related to stomach digestion. It is also important to observe the tongue, which is a storehouse for diagnostic information. In general, over-red, over-pale, dryness, or cracking in the middle of the tongue suggests some form of imbalance of different body systems. Similarly, we can diagnose based on listening and smelling. Is your own talking voice strong or weak? Is your breath rough or light? Do bad odors emanate from the body, for example, bad breath or smelly urine?

We know that eyes are related to liver, ears to kidney, nose to lung, lips to spleen and tongue to heart. We also know that emotions are related to our energy systems. Anger hurts the liver system, sadness impairs the lung, over joy shocks the heart, fear stresses the kidney and over thinking hurts the spleen.

When the kidney is imbalanced, our bodes' defense systems signal a dysfunction. The ear is simply one of our kidney signals. If your kidney meridian is weak, you tend to be hearing-sensitive, have ringing in the ears, fear becomes an overpowering emotion, you lack confidence and lose your decision-making powers. If we don't consider the body as an interconnected, whole system, we may see it isolated by different parts. We may have to see heart specialists, then come back to see a lung specialist, then go to a psychologist for counseling, then see a bone specialist and arthritis specialist, with each doctor seeing only a part of us, much like the aforementioned blind men looking at an elephant without the benefit of the whole picture.

Your condition could start with rheumatic fever, later develop into a heart murmur, years later develop into heart failure, kidney failure and water in the lung. Thus, over time, one small symptom can develop into serious life-threatening diseases.

A group of seemingly unrelated symptoms may actually come from the same root cause. One may feel dryness and redness in the eyes, irritability and anger, headaches, weariness, high cholesterol and blood pressure. All these symptoms can be associated with the yin and yang imbalance of the liver. If we treat the root cause of the imbalance, all symptoms will disappear. However, if we treat each symptom separately—painkillers for headache, eye drops for irritated eyes, physical therapy for back pain, pills for high blood pressure—each medicine will do its job to suppress the symptoms one by one.

Now we as the commanders have shut down the defense system soldiers who tried to report the enemy invaders. We completely disabled the signals! The enemy is already in our castle; the true root cause (an imbalance in our liver) is growing stronger and stronger. Finally, it becomes too late for us to do anything but surrender.

Many recent discoveries confirm the holistic approach of Traditional Chinese Medicine. For example, in her book *The Fat Flush Plan*, nutritionist Ann Louise Gittleman presents a breakthrough diet plan that focuses on cleansing of toxins in the liver—a system fundamental to metabolic efficiency. She writes, "Your liver is a workhorse that can even regenerate its own damaged cells. However, it is not invincible. When it lacks essential nutrients or when it is overwhelmed by toxins, it no longer performs as it should. Hormone imbalances may develop. Fat may accumulate in the liver and then just under the skin or in other organs. Toxins build up and get into your bloodstream."

Among the signs of a toxic liver Gittleman names are:

- Weight gain, especially around the abdomen

- Cellulite

- Abdominal bloating

- Indigestion

- High blood pressure

- Elevated cholesterol

- Fatigue

- Mood swings

- Depression

- Skin rashes

5.2.2   The PingLongevity ™ Eight Treasure Method

There is a simple way to practice TCM based on yin-yang and the five-element theory. The new method treats the fundamental imbalance and weakness of the energy meridian systems rather than the specific diseases. It claims that once the fundamental system is back to optimal condition, disease disappears and can be prevented. The theory focuses on the five fundamental energy meridian systems: heart, lung, liver, kidney and spleen. Each of these five systems, when imbalanced, is either too low in yin and thus too high in yang, or vice versa. We need only eight herbal formulas to address the root causes of diseases. This is a major breakthrough because eight fundamental formulas, instead of thousands, can be used to regenerate the body and return it to its optimal balance.

In Section 1.4.4, we talked about the eight fundamental TCM tests. The tests, combined with eight fundamental formulas, become the Eight Treasure Method, a herbal balancing method of major body meridians and organ systems.

The method comes from the study of the protocols created by top medical scientists and herbalists in China. These formulas are the result of a study of China's 5,000-year-old culture and selections of prescriptions provided by classic texts on medicine and health.

This principle of using the formulas and their associated symptom tests is summarized as follows. All these formulas are time proven and thy are commercially available in the United States and around the world through traditional Chinese herbal stores.

1. Liver One Formula (Xiao Cai Hu Tang Wan)

According to TCM, the liver meridian controls the storage and regulation of blood and vessels. When blood is insufficient, emotion and depression occur. Liver is associated with the tendons and blood vessels. Liver manifests itself in eyes and nails. Liver One deals with liver yin deficiency: not enough blood essence to support the tendons and bones, so symptoms such as weakness of knees and/or blurred and impaired vision occur.

Self-Testing Symptoms:

- Pale complexion
- Dark circles under the eyes
- Anemia
- Scanty menstrual period
- Light menstrual blood color
- Blurred vision
- Dry eyes
- Ophthalmologic problems
- Tight joints

Related diseases: chronic fatigue, anemia, depression.

2. Liver Two Formula (Long Dan Xie Gan Wan)

According to TCM, Liver Two deals with liver yang overacting symptoms. When liver yang is overacting, anger and restlessness occur. Liver Two is associated with blood vessels and gallbladder problems as well as the toxic effects of alcohol, medication, etc. Liver manifests itself in the eyes and nails.

Self-Testing Symptoms:

- Redness, swelling in eyes
- Burning sensation of eyes
- Weak liver function
- Varicose veins

- Bags under the eyes
- Pressure in the eyes
- Trigeminal neuralgia
- Migraine headache
- Menstrual period headache
- Blood pressure above normal
- Irritable, easily angered
- High-pitched ringing in ears
- Urine yellow, scant, burning
- Vertigo, bloating, shaking
- Bloated or full feeling in chest
- Acid reflex, burping
- Tenderness below the ribs
- Cholesterol above normal
- Difficult to concentrate
- Attention deficiency in children
- Gallbladder inflammation
- Dry mouth
- Bitter taste in mouth
- Metallic taste in mouth

Related diseases: high blood pressure, high cholesterol, ADD, anxiety.

3. Kidney One Formula (Jin Kui Shen Qi Wan)

According to traditional Chinese medicine, the kidney yang is for aging, reproduction and growth. Its meridian dominates human reproduction and development, governs water metabolism, produces bone marrow to nourish the brain and dominates bones. It relates to the emotions of fear and determination. It manifests itself in tooth, ear, hair, genitals and the anus. Kidney One is associated with the yang aspect of the kidney meridian.

Self-Testing Symptoms:

- Cold hands or feet
- Incontinence or frequent urination
- Low libido, impotence
- Unable to reach orgasm
- Seminal emission, premature ejaculation, infertility

- Edema and swelling of legs
- Catch colds easily, which can turn into asthma
- Loose stool
- Early morning bowel movement
- Low back pain and backache
- Early menopause
- Fear, tension and stress
- Dream-disturbed sleep
- Shortness of breath and tiredness
- Urinary tract, prostate problems
- Urinate many times at night
- Low immune system
- Pale tongue

Related diseases are: early aging, delayed growth for children.

4. Kidney Two Formula (Liu Wei Di Huang Wan)

According to traditional Chinese medicine, the kidney yin is the basic lubricant fluid in the body. It nourishes organ tissue, bones, and the brain. It relates to the emotion of fear and determination. It manifests itself in tooth, ear, hair, genitals and the anus. Kidney Two deals with the yin aspect of the kidney meridian. Kidney Two is associated with the balance of hormones (e.g., menopause, night sweats, internal heat).

Self-Testing Symptoms:

- Night or afternoon sweating
- Heat/burning in hands, feet
- Sweaty palms
- Anxiety, nervousness
- Decreased memory
- Loose teeth

- Hot flashes, red cheeks, night sweats

- Red flush/rash on face

- Burning and scanty urine

- Hair loss or early graying

- Internal heat, desire cold fluids

- Early ejaculation (male)

- Irregular menstruation (female)

- Deep red tongue

- Low back, waist soreness and weakness

- Joint and bone weakness

- Ear ringing or hearing loss

- Insomnia

- Dizziness

- Scanty menstrual period

- Weight loss

- Canker sore, tongue soreness

Related diseases: sex hormone deficiency.

5. Heart Formula (Sheng Mai San)

According to TCM, the heart meridian governs blood and chi (energy). Blood flows through this meridian under the power of heart chi. If a person is full of vigor, blood circulates smoothly to transport nutrients to all parts of the body. The heart controls mental activities. Mental disorders arise when the heart is injured. The condition of the heart meridian manifests itself in the tongue.

Self-Testing Symptoms:

- Having appetite with no taste

- Pale or purple tongue

- Pale face

- Mental tiredness, sighs often/ feels despair

- Irregular heartbeat, palpitation

- Cold sweat

- Blue lips

- Shallow voice, no energy when speaking

- Short of breath, less energy

- Spontaneous perspiration

- Restless mind, insufficient sleep, multiple dreams

- Forgetfulness, memory loss

- Insomnia

6. Spleen Formula (Bu Zhong Yi Qi Wan)

According to traditional Chinese medicine, the spleen meridian connects to the stomach, governs transportation and transformation of food, and dominates muscles and limbs. An impaired spleen function results in poor digestion and absorption of nutrients. It manifests itself in the mouth (appetite, taste) and lips (pale, swollen).

Self-Testing Symptoms:

- Poor digestion and absorption
- Reduced appetite
- Morning loose stools, diarrhea
- Abdominal distension, heavy sensation
- Leaky gut
- Physical/mental tiredness

- Pale lips and tongue
- Heavy menstrual bleeding
- Muscle pain and weakness
- Tooth marks on the edge of tongue
- Swollen limbs
- Weak muscles

7. Lung Formula (Yang Yin Qing Fei Wan)

According to traditional Chinese medicine, the lung formula deals with lung yin deficiency. The lung meridian dominates the chi of the whole body, controls respiration, nourishes skin and hair and regulates water passageways. It relates to the emotion of sadness and anxiety. It manifests itself in the nose.

Self-Testing Symptoms:

- Dry cough
- Hoarse and low voice
- Dry mouth
- Pimples, acne
- Nose, throat, trachea discomfort

- Scanty sputum
- Chronic sore throat
- Facial speckles
- Rhinitis, hay fever
- Allergy, asthma, dermatitis, hives, cold

- Skin disorder and rashes
- Psoriasis
- Constipation and dry stool
- Weight loss
- Dry throat
- Afternoon fever

8. Cleansing Formula (Qing Ti Pai Du San)

According to TCM, cleansing formula deals with stagnation of heat in the body due to blockage of chi and blood. Toxins accumulate in the body because of long-term imbalances of the meridians. Toxins also accumulate due to fatty, sugary and excessive food intake and high blood pressure. This formula helps calm an overabundance of yang energy in the heart or lung meridians (yang disease) and stagnation of the spleen meridian (overacting of yang). It detoxifies the blood and digestive tracts.

Self-Testing Symptoms:

- Swollen gums
- Thirst, extreme dry mouth
- Dry, cracked lips
- Craving for cold drinks
- Thick coating, dark red tongue
- Constipation
- Bad breath
- Heartburn, stomach ache
- Acid reflex
- Sloshing sounds in stomach
- Pain in the abdomen
- Full stomach distention
- Foul smelling stool

In summary, the Eight Treasure Method is a breakthrough system, which uses eight formulas to balance the yin and yang aspects of the five major organ meridians: lung, heart, liver, kidney and spleen. Each system is associated with a set of symptoms. A set of Eight Fundamental Tests can identify the imbalance easily. Application of eight rather than thousands of formulas keeps the whole body's systems in perfect balance. A balanced system can effectively heal itself.

Now we can see the beauty of the new method: eight formulas

and eight sets of symptoms for diagnosis instead of thousands. Today, we are bombarded with hundreds of different types of vitamins, herbs and supplements, each one targeted to treat certain symptoms. As we become more health conscious, we want to take them all. But should we? How useful are they? We must get back to the fundamentals and there are only a few fundamental formulas that are truly needed for vibrant health.

> "Almost all symptoms are signals from those deep basic root problems and major organ tissues. If you manage to balance energy in those major meridians and organs, you'll be symptom free and feeling healthy. In my practice, I found that if a person has many complaints, doctors should find the major root causes. Usually those root causes are in the liver, kidney, or digestive system. First, focus on those organs, get them working properly. Most of the symptoms will go away. For example, high blood pressure, high cholesterol, varicose veins, sleep disorders, weight gain, hormone imbalance, depression, fatigue, may all be overcome by balancing one organ meridian, the liver. You'll be surprised. You see great results. You'll also feel vibrant health from the inside out. You'll also feel happy because emotions are led by these organ meridians."
>
> —Dr. Ping

5.3   CHI, ENERGY AND THE MERIDIANS

Traditional Chinese Medicine believes that the body consists of three energies, jing, which is the physical part of the body, chi, the invisible energy flowing through the body, and shen, the mind and spirit. Furthermore, it believes that the mind can drive chi through the meridians, chi can direct the flow of blood through the body.

5.3.1   Is Chi Real?

The question: Is chi a real thing?

A pioneering researcher, the American physiologist Dr. Robert

Wallace, conducted a series of experiments in the '60s and '70s at UCLA that tell us something about chi. Meditators were studied over the span of a few years and their biological and physiological data were recorded, including brain waves, blood pressure and heart rate.

It was discovered that meditators, after only a few minutes of meditation, entered into a state of deep relaxation, with a slower heart rate to decreased oxygen consumption. Metabolic rate was also dramatically reduced. Sleep can also achieve some of the same effects. However, you need at least 4 to 6 hours of sleep instead of just a few minutes of meditation to reach the same state. In addition, sleep drops oxygen consumption by about 16% while meditation drops oxygen consumption twice as much.

Deep in the mountains of China, it is said Taoists spend many hours meditating without sleep and food. This is possible because meditation induces a state much more rejuvenating than sleep, a state of increased chi. Due to their reduced metabolic rate, these meditators need very little food, much like the hibernation state of bears in which the animal can sleep the whole winter without food, slowly burning the fat stored in the body for many months. Dr. Wallace called this "hypometabolic wakefulness."

Another study led by Dr. Wallace measured the meditators' biological age. Biological age is different from chronological age. People with the same chronological age, could have a very different biological age. Biological age is the age at which your biological functions—blood pressure, hearing ability, eyesight, blood sugar, athletic ability—are compared to the average population. A 50-year-old may have a biological age of 30 because he or she functions like an average 30-year-old. Dr. Wallace's study showed that meditators as a group have a much younger biological age, by as much as 20 years.

The study also correlated years of meditation with delayed aging. Each year of meditation took off approximately one year of aging. Therefore, 20-year meditators, as a group average, can have as much as a 20-year younger biological age than their peer group, on the average. It was also shown that the effectiveness of meditation does not change relative to age. Hence, it is never too late to gain the effect. Of course, the right method of meditation is also very important.

A 1986 Blue Cross-Blue Shield Insurance study researched 2,000 meditators in Iowa. It was shown that the meditators as a group were much healthier than the average American population in 17 major diseases (they had 87% less occurrence of severe heart disease and 50% fewer tumors).

One study conducted by Dr. Bernard Grad of McGill University in Canada produced interesting information about healers. Dr. Grad had started his research in "hands-on healing" during the 1960s. It was known that healers could lay their hands over diseased areas of patients without touching and create a healing effect. But it was not clear if it was due to the placebo effect (the power of the mind triggered by the patients' belief system).

Dr. Grad conducted a series of experiments using sick plants as the object of treatment to eliminate the placebo effect. Healers were asked to hold bottles of water during their meditation to treat the water. Then sick plants were watered using plain water and treated water. Plants with treated water showed dramatically better growth and returned to health quickly. The study not only demonstrated the existence of a mysterious energy or chi that is not directly measurable by modern technology, but also showed that water is a very good medium for energy storage. This shows why some healers can treat water and send the water hundreds of miles away to use in treating patients. It also shows the importance of drinking high-energy water, such as spring water, not only for its mineral content, but also for its energy content.

To help you appreciate the effect that chi-gong can exert on the internal energy systems, organs and hormonal and nervous systems, we want to talk about an interesting experiment reported in the pioneering book *Creating Energy Body Sciences* by the famous Chinese physicist Qian Xue San, published in 1989. Scientist and chi-gong master Wang Ja Lin of the Yuanang Human chi-Gong Research Institute of China allowed his own gallbladder to be wired to all sorts of instruments for four months' observation. The experiment compared the physiology of the chi-gong state, the relaxed state and sleeping state. It was found that in the chi-gong state, the gallbladder's secretions are much higher than during the usual rest and sleep states, demonstrating that chi-gong indeed can dramatically alter the course of life. Many other reports show that chi-gong can affect the recovery of muscle strain and change heart rates.

Detailed instructions for entering the chi-gong state are given at the end of this chapter.

5.3.2   The Meridians

TCM believes that chi (energy) flows through 12 principle and 8 extra meridians and another 36 subordinate meridians. Each meridian passes through many acupuncture points, sometimes called energy centers. If chi stagnates through the meridians, blood does not flow freely, spirit disperses and essence is weakened. We must open all meridians to have vibrant health.

Indeed, many scientific experiments have proven such meridians and acupuncture points exist. There have been several studies illustrating the physical detectability of acupuncture points such as radioisotope tracing and low electrical impedance at the acupuncture points.

Du (yang) and Ren (yin) meridians are the most important. Du is a major meridian running on the back of the body. It is a yang energy meridian because it faces the sun when we have our hands on the ground. Ren is a major meridian on the front of the body. It belongs to the yin energy meridian. Du and Ren form a circle, called the "microcosmic orbit." They connect through all major organ systems and main energy centers (acupuncture points).

In Section 5.4, we will talk about a simple method of opening and balancing the energy flows of Du and Ren meridians, or the microcosmic orbit, as well as the energy centers along the orbit.

What are Du and Ren meridians and the major energy centers on them?

The Ren meridian has 24 acupuncture points along the front of the body. The following figure shows the points and the meridians.

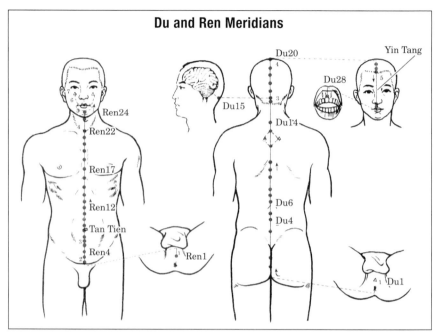

Du and Ren Meridians

Courtesy of Cheng Xinnong, *Chinese Acupuncture and Moxibustion.*

The major acupuncture points are:

Ren1 (Huiyin)—Located midpoint between the anus and the penis or the vagina. This important energy point is called the "Gate of Life." It is the center point of yin energy in the body.

Ren4 (Guanyuan)—Located about midway between the naval and the pubic bone, about $1^1/_2$ inches deep. This energy center is also called the "Ovarian Palace" (for woman) or the "Sperm Palace" (for man).

Tan Tien—Also referred to as lower Tan Tien, this is technically not a point on the Ren meridian, yet it is a most important chi-gong energy center. Located approximately $1^1/_2$ inches inside the naval. *Tan* in Chinese means "pill" (of immortality); *Tien* means "field." Therefore, this is the energy field where the potent chi is collected. It is likened to the furnaces where gold is refined. The ancients believed that if our energy is highly refined through years of meditation, the chi will be strong enough for us to reach immortality.

Ren12 (Zhongwan)—Located halfway between the sternum and the navel, also referred to as middle Tan Tien. This point is sometimes called the solar plexus. It controls spleen, adrenal, pancreas and stomach.

Ren17 (Tanzhong)—Located between the nipples, a very important point, referred to as the heart center. The center relates to rejuvenation of love and joy. It controls the heart and lung.

Ren22 (Tiantu)—Located in the center of the suprasternal fossa (at the throat). This throat energy center relates to thyroid and parathyroid glands and regulates cough and asthma.

Ren24 (Chengjiang)—Located in the depression in the center of the mentolabial groove (between the lower lip and the chin). This is where the Ren meridian ends.

Now let's talk about the Du meridian and the major energy centers. The Du meridian starts at Du1 (Changqiang) and runs through D4 (Mingmen), Du6 (Jizhong), Du14 (Dazhui), Du15 (Yamen), Du20 (Baihui), Yin Tang, and ends at Du28 (YinJiao).

Du1 (Changqiang)—Located midway between the tip of the coccyx and the anus. Called the passage to the door of life and death, this point is where the Ren meridian interacts with the Du meridian. Energy from the Ren must transverse through this point to the Du meridian. If it is not open, energy is lost.

Du4 (Mingmen)—Located opposite the navel on the spine. *Ming* in Chinese means "life" and *men* means "gate." So this is the life gate, where kidney chi is concentrated. Kidney is where the prenatal chi is stored. The left kidney is yang, pertaining to the father and the right kidney is yin, pertaining to the mother. Mingmen is the integration of yin and yang. It is one of the most important points in the body.

Du6 (Jizhong)—Located opposite the solar plexus (R12) on the spine. It relates to the adrenal gland, controlling the response of fight or flight, blood sugar and sodium balance.

Du14 (Dazhui)—Located below the seventh cervical vertebra approximately at shoulder level (the big bone on the neck). It controls cough, asthma, neck pain and back stiffness.

Du20 (Baihui)—Also called the crown, located above the mid-brain. Taoists believe that the spirit enters us in the womb through the crown and it leaves from the crown when we die. The crown is open on newborns (the soft spot on the head) and gradually closes as we age, closing the connection between humans and heaven. Advanced chi-gong requires reopening the crown.

Yin Tang—At the midpoint between the eyebrows, approximately 2 inches inside. This is a very important point, not officially a point on the Du meridian. It is referred to as the original cavity of the spirit, or the third eye, where the spirit sits in the advanced stage of chi-gong. It is a master center, regulating the pituitary and the pineal glands, controlling many life-force functions.

Du28 (YinJiao)—At the junction of the gum and the frenulum of the upper lip. This is the end of the Du meridian.

Microcosmic orbit, which is considered the primary body energy meridians, starts at Tan Tien and ends at Tan Tien. It follows the path of Tan Tien, Ren4, Ren1, Du1, Du4, Du6, Du14, Du20, Yin Tang, Ren22, Ren17, Ren12, Tan Tien. Note that the natural flow of yin meridians (such as Ren) goes downward and the flow of yang meridians (such as Du) goes upward.

5.4   THE CHI-GONG METHOD OF ENERGY BALANCING

As we discussed in Section 5.3, the human body forms its own microcosm, which is connected with the macrocosm of the universe. Chi in the human body travels through the meridians to support the life force in each cell of the body, and at the same time the chi exchanges with the external energies in the universe. When all meridians are open, chi can flow easily. Diseases cannot be accumulated. Energy is transported to all parts of the body. Energy is also absorbed through energy centers/acupuncture points from the outside. When the meridians are blocked, we get into trouble.

Chi-gong is a form of meditation. It is a way to train the body, mind and spirit into a state of complete stillness. When at the extreme of stillness (extreme yin), movement (initial yang) occurs. This movement is the chi in the body running through meridians as well as internal organs. Thus through chi-gong, we can open up all our meridian systems. We can also balance our systems.

Chi-gong is a difficult art because it is dependent on the individual's own mind and emotions. Everyone is so different. That's why Taoist masters talk about "self perception" to be able to "self cultivate." It's like creating a painting: The principles can be easily taught, but becoming a true artist requires self-cultivation.

There are many branches of chi-going, each claiming its own superiority. In fact, all roads may lead to one end point at the highest level of skill. The point here is that practitioners rise above the fray and focus on self-cultivation.

Here's the basic principle of opening the entire microcosmic orbit:

Microcosmic Orbit Chi-Gong:

Basic Positions:

Referring to Section 5.3.2 for all the acupuncture points, start in a sitting position or lotus position, with Du20 (crown) and Ren1 (Huiyin) vertically aligned. Rest both hands on the lap, men with left hand under right hand, left thumb in the right palm, and right thumb pressing on the back of left hand between thumb and index finger. Women use the opposite side. Slightly close the eyes. Touch the soft palate with the tongue to connect the Du and Ren meridians. This is similar to connecting two electrical circuits.

Breathe in and out very slowly, continuously and lightly. Inhale into the lower belly, relaxing the belly muscles and then filling the lung. The mind is completely empty. Continue this throughout the exercise.

The universe is so still. Nothing is moving. You're a part of the universe. You're totally dissolved into it.

Opening Energy Centers:

When you are still and empty, you can move your concentration slightly to the Tan Tien point. Practice for several days or whatever length of time until you can feel sensation (such as warm, numbness, tingling or vibration). When the Tan Tien is open, continue to open other points one at a time.

Move concentration to open R4, Ren1, Du1, Du4, Du6, Du14, Du20, Yin Tang, Ren22, Ren17, Ren12, Tan Tien, consecutively and respectively. Don't leap frog points until they are completely open.

Always finish each session by moving your focus back to the Tan Tien, accumulating chi and storing it there. It is risky to let chi stagnate at other points, especially points on the chest and the head. Care must be taken to return the energy to the Tan Tien.

Circling the Microcosmic Orbit:

Once all energy centers on the microcosmic orbit (Du and Ren meridians) are open, you can use one breath to draw the energy all the way from Hui Yin through the Du meridian up to the crown, and then breathe out to send the chi down through Ren meridian back to the Tan Tien. While your concentration is passing each point, you will feel the chi stirring inside. Thus each breath in and out completes an entire circle of the microcosmic orbit.

Yang Emerging from Extreme Yin:

As your practice is more mature and your microcosmic orbit becomes completely open, you do not have to concentrate through each point and use the mind to circulate the energy on the orbit. As soon as you get into the chi-going state of extreme stillness and emptiness, chi will automatically stir up and flow through your entire body.

Ending Position:

Always end the session by moving your attention back to the Tan Tien.

Practice every day for at least 30 minutes. As you become more experienced, you can reach a chi-gong state at any time, in meetings, waiting in line, sitting at a dinner table, watching TV. Chi-gong becomes part of you and your life and is not limited to your practice time. Continued sessions keep your main meridians balanced and open, accumulate chi and make you stronger and healthier.

With open meridians and energy centers, you will feel extremely comfortable when performing chi-gong. It's a feeling of intoxication that you don't want to end. You will feel every cell of your body breathing, opening and closing. You will feel as if your physical form is disappearing. You will immerse with the vast universe. You will co-exist with the infinite energy source of the universe. Your microcosm will merge with the macrocosm of heaven and earth.

5.5   SUMMARY

We summarize the PingLongevity™ Energy Balance in the following ways:

- An imbalance of energy meridians can be the root cause of many symptoms and diseases. We all have imbalances in our energy systems because we are constantly pushed out of equilibrium due to daily challenges of living. The effects of imbalance accumulate. Longer-term imbalances will shut off energy centers and block meridians. Chinese medicine believes that many diseases are a result of the accumulation of imbalance. Imbalances build little by little, escaping our awareness until they become uncontrollable, when they can result in serious diseases, like cancer.

- The PingLongevity™ Eight Treasure Method is a way to use eight fundamental TCM formulas to balance the yin and yang of the five major organ meridians (i.e., heart, lung, spleen, kidney, and liver), by using a set of symptom tests. You can start by concentrating on the formula where you have a severe symptom. You can also take a formula where you have two or three less severe symptoms. Use the herbs to rebalance the system for 100 days to rejuvenate all the cells of the body back to balance. These herbal formulas have been known for hundreds of years and are available from most Chinese herbal medicine stores.

• You may also use the microcosmic orbit chi-gong method to open and balance energy meridians. Try to perform this every day for at least 30 minutes. Make it part of your daily life so you can gradually be able to reach the chi-gong state at will.

Now we've completed our work on the energy plane, so we can move on to the spiritual plane.

CHAPTER 6

Preserve Spirit Energy

We frequently travel to remote places, such as the Taoist sacred mountains in China, the longevity town Vilcabamba in Ecuador, remote villages of Cambodia and to visit the Masai tribe in East Africa to study their lifestyle, diseases, longevity and spirituality. Typically, they live a very simple life.

Take the Masai for example. People there spend the day herding cattle. While their cattle have good grazing, the people are bathed with the cosmic light and energy. They don't have cravings because they have everything they need. They eat the most nutritious meals —the most pollution-free organic live cow's blood, live milk and occasionally roasted beef. They weave their own fabric that is so colorful and soft on the skin. There are no bars or clubs, but they chant and dance together happily for the simple joy of it. They live in small nomadic huts, sufficient for sleeping. They're the happiest and healthiest people we've seen as we travel around the world studying local cultures and lifestyles.

Just a few hours' drive from the Masai lands in Kenya, we get to the big city of Nairobi, and in a few hours' flight, we are in the cosmopolitan capital, Paris, where our minds are filled with the hustle and bustle.

What is the purpose of our busy-ness? Fame, power, wealth, sex, liquor, drugs, fun and other indulgences? It made us think of what our tai-chi master told us:

"We are born naked with nothing and we die naked, too. We can take nothing with us."

—NANJIE HO, GRAND MASTER

While we are envious of the Masai, we do not choose to live with them. We still enjoy much of what we have in the modern world. What if we could have both worlds simultaneously? All of humankind would be much more spiritual!"

Aging and disease are due to two major fundamental causes: the depletion of vital essence (such as semen, blood, enzymes, hormones, body fluids) and the leakage of spirit energy through emotions and stress. When both essence and spirit energy are reduced, the life-sustaining chi is weakened. However, before puberty, neither leak is substantial. Therefore, the body builds itself toward becoming a higher energy being. Between birth and age 16, the human system is in negative entropy (Chapter 10). Negative entropy indicates a system moving toward more and more organization. A more-organized system has more long-lasting potential. After puberty, we are in positive entropy as we move toward aging and a deteriorating energy potential due to the two deadly leaks of essence and spirit.

This chapter will discuss how to stop the spiritual energy leakage and is the first chapter to deal with our spiritual energy plane. In healing our bodies, spiritual healing is superior and immortal, energy healing is next, food healing is excellent and promotes long life, natural herb healing is good and chemical/surgery healing is the last resort.

6.1   THE STRESSFUL LIFE

We live in a world that grows busier and busier. We evolved from the very slow pace of life in small villages or tribes to modern cosmopolitan life. People in remote tribes are not bombarded with news on television, the Internet, iPods, Facebook and iPads. They have simple social standards, simple jobs, mostly related to the basic activities of making a living (hunting, farming, etc.), and a simple life. Money is not that useful. Even if they had money, there is nowhere to spend it. Fame is confined to a very small circle. Lust is not within the social/tribal standard. Power is absolute from the tribal leaders. There are simply not enough things for people to crave and fight for. Time flows slowly. After dark, there is no electricity. People sit around chatting and watching stars. The mind works slowly because speed is not needed. As long as people can make a basic living, there is nothing else available for them to seek.

In contrast, in modern life there is so much to be desired. We want more money, a bigger house, better cars, vacations, travel, better jobs, career advancement, power and fame and to indulge in sex, food and play. The efficient information flow due to modern technology (newspapers, transportation, Internet, database, TV, radio) has overpowered us with all kinds of opportunities to seek and crave more. Every minute we are presented with opportunities, which lure us to work harder. We hear news of an economic slowdown and crank up our computers to sell stocks. We see ads on the Internet for jobs that give us hope for better-paying positions and suddenly find ourselves in the job-interviewing process. We hear about a sale at a supermarket and hurry out to buy. We become angry when co-workers take credit for our work. We are sued because others simply want to make some extra dollars. We get ticketed for speeding, angry with our car dealers and anxious when the lawn and trees are dying because the sprinkler is broken.

But even this is not enough excitement, so we watch movies that are suspenseful, violent, sexual and highly emotional. All of this stimulates emotional stress. There is just too much! Every minute of our lives is occupied. How many times are our brain cells buzzing, compared with people in primitive tribes? We'd bet over a million times. That would make an interesting research project.

Here are some statistics on modern stress, according to Kessler et al, National Comorbidity Survey Replication, *Archives of General Psychiatry:*

- Major depressive disorders affect approximately 14.8 million American adults, or about 6.7 percent of the U.S. population ages 18 and older in a given year

- An estimated 26.2 percent of Americans ages 18 and older—about one in four adults—suffer from a diagnosable mental disorder in a given year.

- Symptoms of dysthymic disorder (chronic, mild depression) must persist for at least two years in adults (one year in children) to meet criteria for the diagnosis. Dysthymic disorder affects approximately 1.5 percent of the U.S. population age 18 and older in a given year.

- Bipolar disorder affects approximately 5.7 million American adults, or about 2.6 percent of the U.S. population ages 18 and older in a given year.

- Approximately 40 million American adults ages 18 and older have an anxiety disorder, about 18.1 percent of people in this age group in a given year.

- Approximately 6 million American adults ages 18 and older have panic disorder, about 2.7 percent of people in this age group in a given year.

- Approximately 2.2 million American adults age 18 and older have obsessive compulsive disorder (OCD), about 1.0 percent of people in this age group in a given year.

- Approximately 6.8 million American adults have generalized anxiety disorder (GAD), or about 3.1 percent of people ages 18 and over, in a given year.

- Approximately 15 million American adults age 18 and over have social phobia, about 6.8 percent of people in this age group in a given year.

No doubt we are living in a world that is exciting, but stressful, especially if we don't know how to handle our stress. It is impossible for most of us to have the luxury of retirement or semi-retirement or to even to slow the pace of our lives to preserve our health.

We mentioned earlier the ways life insurance companies set their premiums. Insurance companies have to do a good job of estimating the length of life and the risk of death because that is how they make money. One aspect of the premium estimate is to classify people into occupational categories. It's interesting that the following are listed as life-extending occupations: symphony orchestra conductor, scientist and mathematician, university professor, successful creative artist, U.S. government employee. As you can see, these occupations happen to be ones with less stress as compared to corporate executives, athletes, dotcom company employees, small business owners or politicians. Those with less stress can immerse themselves in their specialties (such as math), their enjoyment (orchestra conductor) and their unconscious mind creativity (artists), highly concentrating their minds on a single subject in which they can by and large forget about things happening around them. These are usually jobs not involving stressful deadlines or complex political maneuvers or power struggles.

Growing emotional distress is a phenomenon spanning thousands of years of human evolution. It is not a new problem, except that today it is more intensified.

An interesting dialog can be found in *The Yellow Emperor's Classic of Medicine*. The following dialog took place between the Huang Di and his advisor Qi Bo:

> "Huang Di asked, 'I've heard that in the days of old, everyone lived 100 years without showing the usual signs of aging. In our time, however, people age prematurely, living only 50 years. Is this due to a change in the environment, or is it because people have lost the correct way of life?'
>
> Qi Bo replied, 'In the past, people practiced the Tao, the Way of Life. They understood the principle of balance, of yin and yang, as presented by the transformation of the energies of the universe. Thus, they formulated practices such as Dao-in, an exercise combining stretching, massaging and breathing to promote energy flow. They also meditated to help maintain and harmonize themselves with the universe. They ate a balanced diet at regular times, arose and retired at regular hours, avoided overstressing their bodies and minds and refrained from overindulgence of all kinds. They maintained well-being of body

and mind; thus, it is not surprising that they lived over 100 years.

These days, people have changed their way of life. They drink wine as though it were water, indulge excessively in destructive activities, drain their jing—the body's essence that is stored in the kidneys—and deplete their chi. They do not know the secret of conserving their energy and vitality. Seeking emotional excitement and momentary pleasures, people disregard the natural rhythm and order of the universe. They fail to regulate their lifestyle and diet and sleep improperly. So it is not surprising that they look old at 50 and die soon after.

The accomplished ones of ancient times advised people to guard themselves against gu zei feng, disease-causing factors. On the mental level, one should remain calm and avoid excessive desires and fantasies, recognizing and maintaining the natural purity and clarity of the mind. When internal energies are able to circulate smoothly and freely and the energy of the mind is not scattered but is focused and concentrated, illness and disease can be avoided.

Previously, people led a calm and honest existence, detached from undue desire and ambition; they lived with an untainted conscience and without fear. They were active, but never depleted themselves. Because they lived simply, these individuals knew contentment, as reflected in their diet of basic but nourishing goods and attire that was appropriate to the season but never luxurious. Since they were happy with their position in life, they did not feel jealousy or greed. They had compassion for others and were helpful and honest, free from destructive habits. They remained unshakable and unswayed by temptations and they were able to stay centered even when adversity arose. They treated others justly, regardless of their level of intelligence or social position."

—THE YELLOW EMPEROR'S CLASSIC OF MEDICINE

6.2   MODERN SCIENCE'S VIEW OF STRESS

Modern science looks at emotion, craving, and desire from the point of view of stress. There is no doubt that severe emotion creates stress and craving and desire for things creates emotion.

There is a strong link between emotion and hormones. The pituitary is the master gland of hormones, sitting behind the eyes inside the brain. It controls the release of many hormones, including growth hormones. When emotions arise, hormones are affected and a series of physiological responses occurs. When you are fed up with a person who is seeking a loving relationship, you immediately are "turned off" (of all your sexual hormones). Many women, for example, find that being anxious or upset may delay menstruation.

It works the other way also. When hormones change, emotions rise. For example, menopausal women or an andropausal men, when their sex hormones experience dramatic imbalance, experience mood swings and depression.

6.2.1 The Fight or Flight Response

In our autonomic nervous system, the sympathetic nervous system's response to stress is often referred to as "fight, flight or freeze," while the parasympathetic nervous system is sometimes called "rest and digest."

There are two major hormones involved in stressful situations. The sympathetic nervous system is regulated by the hormone adrenaline and the parasympathetic nervous system by acetylcholine. When we experience fear, anger or strong emotional reactions, adrenaline is released, putting us into a state of "fight or flight." When we are out of an "emergency" state and relaxed, acetylcholine kicks in, putting us into a "rest and digest" mode. The sympathetic and parasympathetic nervous systems complement each other, much like the gas and the brakes on a car.

When the body is in a state of stress, adrenaline works hand-in-hand with another hormone, cortisol. Adrenaline works in the short term, while cortisol has momentum and works in the long term. The primary functions of cortisol in stress are to increase blood sugar through gluconeogenesis and suppress the immune system.

Just when your level of adrenaline starts coming down, the levels of cortisol rise. Even though it builds slowly, cortisol also takes a long time to return to normal. If you are constantly engaging in activities that stimulate adrenaline, your levels of cortisol will slowly increase. In a sense, you can think of cortisol as a measure of the weighted average of your recent levels of adrenaline. The combined effects of adrenaline and cortisol are to:

- Make the heart beat faster and harder to pump blood, increasing blood flow to the muscles, lungs, and brain;

- Raise blood pressure by restricting blood vessels near the surface of the body and the gut so that more blood can be supplied to the heart;

- Stimulate the lungs to breathe harder to supply more oxygen for higher fuel burning;

- Release more blood cells, which increases the blood's ability to transport oxygen;

- Cause the immune system to redirect white blood cells to the skin, bone marrow and lymph nodes, where injury or infection are most likely to occur;

- Shut down the digestive process and many other temporarily "unnecessary" body functions;

- Raise the blood sugar level by accelerating the conversion of glycogen stored in the liver and the muscles, in order to prepare the extra energy required in a fight and flight situation;

- Dilate the pupils, dry the mouth and cause sweating.

6.2.2   The Detrimental Impact of Chronic Stress

Now let's think about the effects of prolonged stress.

When humans all lived primitively, people could escape from dangerous situations and return to a state of relaxation. However, in today's environment, we hardly can escape from the constant stress. Many of us spend long workdays in stressful environments competing in the market economy, doing good work, earning promotions, making more money and achieving recognition. We then spend our dinnertime socializing in order to build relationships with people important to our work or to get a deal done with business partners. Before we go to bed, we take care of our children and family chores. The next day, we are in the same cycle again. Modern life has turned our stress hormone from an occasional stressor to a constant one.

The long-term effect of stress is more related to the hormone cortisol. It is sometimes called the sugar hormone because it is responsible for raising blood sugar levels. There are several hormones that elevate blood sugar level, but there is only one that reduces sugar levels: insulin. When the sugar level is constantly raised, insulin becomes deficient or the ability for insulin to act upon cells becomes deficient. In such a case, diabetes can and will result. Under stress, cortisone stimulates the conversion of protein to blood sugar in order to increase the fuel to fight the stressful situation. That protein is mostly derived from the breakdown of muscle tissue; thus, chronically elevated cortisone leads to accelerated muscle reduction. Furthermore, it is also a major cause of bone mass loss. Cortisol is basically a catabolic (the process of breaking down things in the body) hormone that tears down tissue and bones in order to raise the blood sugar level.

Medically, we use cortisone for many emergency situations. It can be life saving for people with asthma in the midst of a severe breathing crisis or for people with severe allergies called anaphylaxis. In many cases, the use of cortisone or a cortisone-like medicine will immediately relieve the emergency situation. This is because cortisone works to reduce inflammation. However, a constant release of cortisone from the body due to stressful situations or the intake of externally administered cortisone is actually immuno-suppressive and toxic to the thymus—the master organ responsible for immune functions. In addition, chronic high levels of cortisone interfere with the building of muscles and cartilage, damage neurons leading to memory loss and can cause poor brain function. Some theories of female adult acne also place the blame on cortisone for the aging effects of skin due to a period of prolonged stress.

For the body to produce cortisone, it uses the main precursor hormone pregnenolone to make glucocorticoids. But the same precursor hormone is also used to make DHEA, the antioxidant hormone, as well as other important anti-aging hormones such as progesterone and testosterone. Thus, constant stress resulting in constant production of cortisone reduces the production of other very useful hormones. Elevated cortisone also means lower production of the thyroid hormones, which are so important for the regulation of metabolism. This further accelerates the aging process.

DHEA, widely believed as a hormone to combat oxidants and keep the body healthy and young, is our built-in defense against excess cortisone. In fact, most of the benefit of DHEA can be explained in terms of its role as an inhibitor of the biological actions of corticosteroids. Some anti-aging doctors believe that the ratio between cortisone and DHEA is a good measure of aging. Under stress, the production of cortisone is higher, whereas the production of DHEA is lower. Thus, chronic stress raises the ratio and accelerates aging.

Interestingly in men, there is a clear antagonistic relationship between insulin and DHEA. Lowering insulin (whether through carbohydrate-restricted diet or through insulin-lowering drugs creates dramatically higher DHEA levels. In both sexes, meditation not only lowers cortisone, but also raises DHEA.

Why does all this stress matter? A chronic high stress hormone level causes abnormal responses in the body: high blood pressure, high blood sugar, restricted circulation of blood to the surface of the body, the shutdown of the digestive process and other body functions and impairs the immune system. Studies have shown many chronic diseases linked to stress. Below are just some major ones:

• Immune system: A study, by Dr. O'Leary published on Psychological Bulletin in 1990, observed students in an academic environment during exam time and found that the level of T-cells and responses to mitogens was lower, and there was a higher self-reported occurrence of health problems, such as upper respiratory-tract infections.

• Neurodegenerative diseases: "Chronic stress can intensify inflammation and increase a person's risk for developing central nervous system infections, neurodegenerative diseases, like multiple sclerosis (MS), and other inflammatory diseases, say researchers presenting at the 115th Annual Convention of the American Psychological Association (APA), Aug. 17, 2007.

- Cardiovascular diseases: "In a six-year study of 860 people over 65, those with the highest levels of cortisol had a five-fold risk of death from cardiovascular disease." (*BBC News*, September 10, 2010)

- Diabetes: An animal study, led by Dr. Mark P. Mattson, from Princeton University, "indicates that the cognitive impairment that can occur in people with diabetes appears to result from high levels of the stress hormone cortisol." (*Reuters Health*, February 19, 2008)

- Obesity: "'Increasing levels of stress accurately predicted increased body mass index (BMI), increased weight gain, increased caloric intake and higher dietary fat intake,' concludes lead author, Paula Rhode, PhD, a clinical psychologist and professor of preventive medicine and public health at the University of Kansas. Stress and depression predicted 26% of the variance in weight gain and 29% of the increase in BMI." (*American Diabetes Association News*, January 2006)

- Depression: "Harvard Medical School researchers have shown that chronic exposure to a stress hormone directly leads to symptoms of depression." (*Red Herring*, April 16, 2006)

- Cancer: "According to a study published in September in the journal *Cancer Research*, metastasis—the spread of cancer cells to other organs– and the effects of stress is a major factor in mortality rates for breast cancer." (October 1, 2010, *Daily Bruin*, UCLA)

- Infertility: "It's long been suspected that stress can affect a woman's ability to get pregnant. But now for the first time ever, scientists have found some concrete evidence that stressed out women have a harder time conceiving." (*NBC*, September 30, 2010)

- Autism: "Some of the symptoms of the autistic condition Asperger's Syndrome, such as a need for routine and resistance to change, could be linked to levels of the stress hormone cortisol, suggests new research led by the University of Bath." (*Medical News Today*, April 1, 2009)

- Gastrointestinal diseases: "Certain stressful life events have been associated with the onset or symptom exacerbation in some of the most common chronic disorders of the digestive system, including functional gastrointestinal disorders (FGD), inflammatory bowel disease (IBD), gastro-esophageal reflux disease (GERD) and peptic ulcer disease (PUD)." (Dr. Mayer, *Gut*, 2000; 47.)

- The digestive system does not function properly and nutrition is not well absorbed. Blood sugar is high and insulin rises, making us fat and more prone to diabetes. Just note the statistics: from 1990 to 1998, diabetes jumped 33%, 70% in the 30–39 age group, 40% in 40–49 age group, and 31% in 50–59 age group, according to data provided by the Centers for Disease Control and Prevention. By age 50, one in ten Americans have diabetes and many more have a blood sugar level at the high end of the "normal" range defined by the medical professions. Also according to the latest national statistics, 61% of American adults are overweight as defined by a body mass index over 25 (BMI = metric weight divided by the square of metric height).

In summary, chronically elevated adrenaline and cortisol in a stressful lifestyle can have detrimental effects on health.

6.3   THE TCM VIEW OF STRESS

Traditional Chinese Medicine and Taoist sages thousands of years ago recognized stress as having a significant impact on the body.

In the classic *Cultivating Stillness*, written in the era between 220–589 C.E. by Lao Tzu, the father of Taoism, we find the following teaching about human nature, spirit and mind:

"If people can constantly be pure and still, then heaven and earth will return to their places. The spirit tends toward purity, but the mind disturbs it. The mind tends toward stillness but it is opposed by craving. If you are able to control desire, then the mind will be still. Clear the mind and the spirit will be pure. Those who are unable to attain the Tao are those whose minds are not clear and who are still slaves of their emotions. Look into your mind and there is no mind. Look at appearances and appearances have no forms. Gaze at distant objects and objects do not exist. Understand these three modes of cognition and you will see emptiness."

—LAO TZU

In the first sentence of this quote, heaven refers to spirit and earth refers to essence in the microcosm of the human body. In its prenatal state, the two are united. Yin and yang are together. Mind and body are one. This oneness represents the original higher vibrating energy. It stays young and lasts long. In the postnatal state, yin and yang become separated. Life becomes limited. Life now follows the universal energy hypothesis to be discussed in Chapter 10. Therefore, Lao Tzu said that if we can really achieve a state of mind of stillness and emptiness, we can unite the spirit, chi and essence and become immortal. People cannot achieve this due to craving, desire and emotions.

In TCM, there are seven deadly emotions. These are the emotions of overjoy, anger (rage), sadness, pensiveness (overly thoughtful), grief, fear and fright. Each of these emotions is considered harmful to the body's energy systems. They weaken spirit energy. The ancient Chinese believed that the natural leakage of spiritual energy flows upward. Each flush of emotion reduces our spiritual energy reserve. Through a lifelong process of overjoy, anger, sadness, pensiveness, grief, fear and fright, we gradually deplete ourselves of our spiritual energy reserve. Thus we grow older and older, following the path of the law of life. Emotions are also related to the five major organ meridian systems. They block and weaken these systems.

Body, mind and spirit are all connected. For example, heart is the master of spirit. This is very different from Western medicine where the heart is considered merely a blood pump. When a musician's heart is transplanted to a person, the recipient may become more fond of music. When the mind is frustrated, the heart feels uncomfortable. When a person is kind and loving, we often say this person has a good heart. So it is extremely important to realize that emotions, mind and the different parts of the body are connected.

Overjoy is related to heart energy. The expression "dying laughing" means people die during intense laughter because they strike the heart too hard. When overjoyed, the heart needs to pump blood hard to fuel the joy. It scatters the heart energy or chi. Joy at its normal level is healthy. If we have an optimistic outlook on life and are naturally happy and joyful, it warms the heart and cheers the spirit. However, taken to the extreme, it is very harmful and needs to be avoided. Fright is the opposite of overjoy. Fright is due to a sudden change of environment. It strikes the heart. It disturbs the spirit.

Anger is very bad for liver energy. It causes stagnation of chi and blood. We often see people's faces turn blue or white and eyes turn red when they are in extreme rage. We see people shake with rage. The liver is the organ system that manufactures and stores blood. When liver chi is impaired due to anger, then blood and chi circulation is interrupted.

This brings to mind a patient who had periodic headaches. Every few weeks, he would get a sinus infection, sore throat, gum pain, sore eyes and headaches. We discovered that he frequently went through very stressful situations. His temper had built up over time.

When the anger accumulates, it turns into liver yang imbalance, as discussed in the preceding chapter. The extra yang due to anger flares up to cause all the symptoms. In Western medicine, it would be called inflammation. At each outburst of this imbalance, the body fights hard and returns to a state of balance until the accumulation becomes too large again.

Sadness hurts the lung energy. When people are extremely sad, they weep and have difficulty catching their breath. When lung energy is blocked, people usually feel oppressed in the chest and depressed. Excessive grief also impacts the digestive process and injures the lungs. It leads to the stagnation of lung chi, leading to hypofunctioning of internal organs. That is why we see people with excessive grief having difficulty breathing, listlessness and depression.

> "A few years ago, I saw a 17-year-old boy who had suffered from severe dry cough for several months nonstop. He got no relief from many medications prescribed by many specialists. When I saw him, after some diagnosis, I found that his symptoms started right after he lost his sister. I knew that it was because of the sadness that impaired his lung function. Besides strengthening his lung function, I also helped regulating his autonomic nervous system. His cough went away in three days."
>
> —DR. PING

Excessive pensiveness injures the spleen. It is said in the ancient Chinese classic *Plain Questions*, "The spleen is the organ that stores intention and shares control of determination. With the heart, it decides everything." The spleen system is also responsible for transporting nutrients and water throughout the body. Thus prolonged excessive pensiveness impairs the digestive system.

Here's a simple experiment: Do some very hard thinking, perhaps working on a problem at work while you're eating dinner. You can feel the impact of overthinking on your digestion. Unfortunately, dining has become one of the important means of conducting business or other high-pressure social events that require hard thinking, taking the mind away from enjoying food.

Fear affects kidney energy, due to hypofunctioning of internal organ systems. It causes nightmares and bad dreams.

The root causes of the seven deadly emotions of overjoy, anger, sadness, pensiveness, grief, fear and fright are usually caused by desire and cravings for power, wealth, fame, food and sex. These desires have been intensified in our materialistic world. For example, there are many opportunities to make money and there are unlimited places to spend money. There is always something to buy. There are more and more things to crave as materialism advances. The Internet, TV, magazines, books and radio lead our emotions in all sorts of directions.

Emotions due to worldly cravings are among the major root causes of poor health and accelerated aging. We'll talk in later sections about ways to reduce such spiritual energy leakage in order to preserve youthfulness.

6.4   STRESS REDUCTION TECHNIQUES

You may now be wondering, if it is possible to avoid all harmful emotions. How can we reduce daily stress? How can we keep adrenaline and cortisone levels reasonably low?

Obviously it is not possible to live in a totally stress-free environment if we want to continue living in this modern world. Most of us choose not to live in caves in the mountains like the ancient sages. We don't always have the luxury of choosing where we want to work. We have to push ourselves hard, or be pushed to work hard. We have to feed our families, drive on smog-filled congested freeways, deal with politics, laws and social standards, all somewhat unnaturally forced upon us. We feel the need to buy brand-name clothing for our kids and strive for better cars, houses, education, restaurants, social status, power, money and fame.

This is how most of us function in busy modern everyday life. We are busier than the bees, stressed to the extreme and we keep building up the pressure.

But, yes, there is a way to experience emotions without depleting our spiritual energy and depriving ourselves of our young vibrant life!

To understand how we can rid ourselves of stress, we must understand the cumulative effect of the body, mind and spirit. Emotional stress is a positive feedback system, and it is an unstable system. In the automatic control theory, a negative control is a stable system. In a negative control system, a reference signal is provided (such as the desired room temperature in the air conditioning control panel). When the output (the actual room temperature) is higher than the desired setting, AC is turned on to lower the temperature. Here the negative control is that the control action is in the opposite direction (lower the temperature) of the actual (higher temperature).

On the other hand, a positive control system is unstable. Its control action is in the same direction of the output. An example of this would be a control that keeps the AC off and the heater on as the room temperature becomes higher and higher than the desired level, until it is too hot in the room. Similarly, stress is also a positive feedback system. The longer we are in a stressful state, the greater the deterioration of our overall spiritual health.

Here is an everyday example: We see a co-worker in a bad mood. He must have had a bad experience—maybe he was passed over for a promotion. Because of it, he looks at everything from a dark side. It now appears to him that everything and everyone is against him. This ever-spiraling elevation of emotional stress can be explained easily through the viewpoint of TCM.

Anger affects your eating and sleeping. It drains energy. It impairs your liver energy system, since anger is the emotion that impairs the liver the most. When the liver is impaired, you become irritable because the liver relates to the emotion of anger and depression. According to the five-element theory, liver is wood. It promotes fire (heart). If liver is weak, heart energy is also impaired. Liver produces blood, and the heart transports blood. When the heart is weak, you become restless and sleepless. Your spirit becomes a wanderer. But heart is fire and it promotes earth (spleen). Therefore heart weakness affects the health of the spleen system. Nutrients cannot be converted and absorbed effectively. You tire easily, both physically and mentally. This makes you more depressed. Spleen is earth and it promotes metal (lung). With the lung system impaired, you fall victim to allergies, flu, colds, coughs and asthma. Your anxiety level is high. Since lung is metal, it promotes water (kidney), so your kidney energy is weakened. You become more hesitant. Therefore, your bones and joints are weak and your marrow is lacking. This is because TCM believes the kidney meridian controls bones, joints and the health of bone marrow. You become impotent and lose hair. As kidney is water, it promotes wood (liver).

You have made one big circle: from chronic anger to liver, to heart, to spleen, to lung, to kidney, back to liver—a destructive circle through all five major organ energy systems. Long-term stress builds up until it destroys your health and depletes your spirit energy.

Therefore, we must learn how to release stress instantaneously. Never let it accumulate. It is far too dangerous to health and longevity.

6.4.1   Chi-Gong Methods

When our bodies are dirty, we wash. When our teeth are dirty, we brush them. When we eat dirty food, we need detoxification to cleanse our blood and digestive tract. When we get fat, we hurry to lose weight. When our bodies contract a bacterial infection, we use antibiotics to flush it out.

All these are nothing compared to the dirtiness of emotional stress, the root cause of declining health. We need a spiritual and mental cleanup to improve health and longevity.

We should be able to sleep well, free of disturbing dreams. We must not let stress accumulate even for one day. A very effective solution is pre-bedtime meditation. This resets the mind and spirit, detoxifies all the emotional stress of the day, calms the mind for a good night's sleep and renews you for the next day. The following is a simple routine. Perform it nightly for 30 minutes before sleep.

Tan Tien Meditation

Start in a sitting position, with Du20 (crown at the top of the head) and Ren1 or Huiyin (Section 5.3.2) vertically aligned. Place feet flat on the floor. Rest both hands on the lap, with left hand under right hand, left thumb in the right palm, and right thumb pressing on the back of left hand between thumb and index finger (women use the opposite hands). Close your eyes. Touch the soft palate with the tongue to connect the Du and Ren meridians, similar to connecting two electrical circuits. Breathe in and out very slowly about 1 to 4 times per minute. Start in the lower belly, filling up toward the lungs. Relax the whole body, every muscle, tendon, ligament, bone. Focus your attention on the Tan Tien (inside the navel). Listen to your breath going in and out. Completely empty the mind— absolutely no thoughts, no form, no imagination. Everything is supernatural through complete immersion into the vast universe.

For more advanced meditation, you may use the following technique:

Chi-Gong State Meditation

Prerequisite: You must first have a completely open microcosmic orbit through the method discussed in Section 5.4 before you practice this method.

Start in a sitting position, with Du20 (crown of the head) and Ren1 or Huiyin (Section 5.3.2) vertically aligned. Place feet flat on the ground or sit cross legged. Close your eyes. Touch the soft palate with the tongue. Breathe in and out, so slow and so light, as though there is no breath. Completely empty the mind—absolutely no thoughts, no form, no imagination. Turn your sight internally, seeing and feeling chi simmering in your entire body, and penetrating every part of your being. Feel your physical boundaries become blurred, expanded and vaporized. The world is so still, and yet, there's a stir of chi everywhere, merging your disappeared physical body with the universe.

When you reach the chi-gong state, your hands will be warm. Your body will be in a harmonious state—chi and blood bring warmth throughout every part of the body. Your mind and spirit will feel so luxuriously comfortable, almost intoxicated, that you won't ever want to leave this state of relaxation.

This turns weak into strong, dispersed into concentrated, degenerated into vibrant, impotent into vital. It reunites the three treasures, the spirit, chi and essence. You must achieve absolute stillness of body (relax) and mind (empty).

When your are finished, gradually take all of the universe,

including all the cosmic energy, rays, chi, lights back to your Tan Tien (inside the naval). Condense it smaller and smaller into the limitation of your physical form and then into the small size of your Tan Tien. Stay in there until you feel settled, and ready to open your eyes.

Note that in advanced practice, you should be able to reach chi-gong state at any moment and place, with any postures. You may be "there" standing in line waiting for cashier, or in a car, or in a meeting. As soon as you want, you may direct yourself into this state. It also does not matter if you have your eyes open or not. At this advanced level, all the forms and postures, anything physical, which many chi-gong masters conventionally teach, because you have surpassed them. Chi-gong is actually so simple in physical form, and yet so complex in terms of your own perception, wisdom, and spirituality.

6.4.2   Compartmentalize Stressful Situations

It's clear from Section 6.2.2, that chronic stress and elevated stress hormones, adrenaline and cortisol are due to a long-term lifestyle of constant stress. Thus, it's very important to make sure that you are not in stressful situations every hour, every day, all the time.

It may not be difficult for you to list your top stressful situations. Make that list. For example, your top three stressful situations may be:

List of Stressors (Example):

- Not having enough time to do everything you need to do

- Workplace politics

- Tight task delivery date at work

- Socializing with co-workers, bosses, customers, suppliers

- Do household chores, kids, grocery, cooking, cleaning

You should also list the top things that relax you.

List of Relaxers (Example):

- Take an after-dinner walk alone or with a partner

- Wondering around electronic stores to see the newest gadgets

- Play golf

- Hiking

- Read a book in a quiet place

- Meditation

- Yoga

Although there's no way to avoid the list of stressors, you must make sure that each day you compartmentalize the stressors within predefined hours. When you are out of the hours, you refuse to think of, or deal with the stress.

Many people cannot do this. For example, they cannot miss an e-mail, or a phone call. They may be bombarded with urgent work-related calls and are replying to e-mails, all the time, even when they are trying to relax. As a result, they are at a high stress level all day long, every day, throughout their lives.

Therefore, the rules of compartmentalization are:

- Make your own list of stressors and relaxers.

- Activities in the list of stressors are restricted to the WORKING SLOTS, the times you designate for working.

- No discussion, emails, phone calls, thoughts related to any activities on the list of stressors are allowed in LEISURE SLOTS (outside of WORKING SLOTS).

- Make the SLOTS as regularly fixed times as possible, so the body gets conditioned to the rhythm.

All of us have our own original nature, very comfortable in one way or another. Some people enjoy social occasions, others don't.

Similarly, some like publicity, being in front of cameras and in the spotlight, while others are more private. Some of us are OK with pressure, such as meeting deadlines, while others don't like pressure at all.

In real life, we sometimes won't be able to choose a job that perfectly fits our nature. Therefore, we have to be a little outside of our original nature in order to be successful in the modern business or social world.

Some of us are innately quiet, but we have to stretch our necks occasionally with public speaking engagements. Some of us like loose casual clothing because it is comfortable, but we have to dress for success by strangling ourselves with neckties and squeezing our feet into hard leather shoes. Some of us don't like a few of our co-workers, but we have to say good things about them and be charming at social dinners. Some of us don't enjoy working too hard but still do it because we think we have to. Some of us don't like having to leash our dogs on the beach, but we have to follow the rule. Some of us like natural milk straight from the cow and fresh-squeezed orange juice, but we cannot find them in the supermarket. They may even be unlawful.

This is the modern world. We are part of it. On one hand, it is great to live in such a world, but on the other, we have to move ourselves away from our natural state in order to live in it. De-naturing ourselves all the time is deadly to our health and longevity. If we can develop an ability to switch between two lives, natured and de-natured, then we can find ways to separate our lives into two segments, two co-existing lives.

Imagine that you are two completely different people every day. On one hand, during working hours you are competitive, hard-working, social, driving—a success in every way. On the other hand, during off hours and weekends, you are a natural person—casual, honest, naïve, yourself, simple, relaxed, slow-paced, easygoing, free-spirited, calm-minded, quiet, unrestricted—the epitome of primitive original nature.

You don't answer cell phones, get onto work computer networks, socialize for the sake of work, do business travel or worry about work. In essence, you have completely separated the two lives. You now can live two lives independently—one in the competitive, worldly, materialistic realm, the other in the still, emotionless, stressless, empty-minded spiritual realm. This is the only way to preserve our spirit, the highest energy source of life. If you can indeed achieve such a state of mind and lifestyle, you can easily reset your stress levels to zero every day. You will find so much more enjoyment in life, the way our natural lives were intended to be.

6.4.3   Adopt the Taoist View of Life

As discussed in Section 6.3, almost all stresses are expressed by the seven deadly emotions, as a result of some sort of craving and desire, for money, power, fame, material goods (house, cars), sex, love and food. Most of the time, you work so hard for things that even if you ultimately get them, you do not really have the time to enjoy them.

How often have we heard about a father who worked hard his entire life, retired at 65, believing his dreams had come true and then died suddenly from a heart attack. Such a pity: a lifetime of accumulation with enjoyment cut short.

We often see old people suffering with degenerative diseases. What is the use of fame, power, money, sex and food if our health cannot be maintained? Many times we see the rich and famous become old and lose their living ability through Alzheimer's disease or a stroke. Sometimes nobody cares about them anymore, not even family members.

We arrive in the world naked. We leave the world naked, too. We bring nothing to the world and we can take nothing with us. The things in our worldly life are both real and perceived.

The real achievement of life is determined by your fate. In Einstein's relativity theory, space and time are relative. Future events can be seen in the present. Thus, in the relative sense, the future events have already been determined. You should try your best to do good work. If something is meant to be yours, it will be yours.

If it is not meant to be yours, it is not going to be yours. If you are rich, it's great. It's meant to be that way. If you are famous, great too. But if you are not, so be it. It is your destiny.

There is an old Chinese saying that, "Man proposes, God disposes." At the end of the Han Dynasty (around 200 A.D.), China was divided into three kingdoms: Shu, Wu, and Wei. There was a deciding battle, which could have helped Shu to unify the entire country if it was won. Shu's commander, through very smart strategy, lured Wei troops into a narrow road deep inside a canyon sandwiched by sharp cliffs. The Shu army then blocked the escape at both ends of the road, and set fire to the whole canyon, shooting arrows and stones at the Wei troops. It seemed the Wei troops had no chance for survival. The commander of Wei, a very talented warrior, facing his entire army being destroyed, sighed emotionally, "It's heaven's intent to terminate me." Suddenly, out of the blue sky, a gusty wind brought a huge rainstorm, which completely extinguished the fire. The Wei troops fought their way out of the canyon and escaped. Later, Wei became stronger and unified the whole country into the Jin Dynasty.

The moral of the story is that although the Shu commander tried his best and did a superior job in strategy, he still could not unite the country. Thus, "Man proposes, God disposes."

We may dream of becoming millionaires overnight, we may want a promotion badly, we may desire the fame of movie stars. But all we need to do is simply our best and hope to attain the best results. Emotion and worry do not help anything if everything is pre-arranged. Many times, emotion does not solve anything but makes you miserable, not just temporarily feeling terrible but permanently marring your health.

There is a pertinent message in the lyrics of "For Now" from the famous Broadway show *Avenue Q* written by Jeff Whitty:

PRINCETON: Why does everything have to be so hard?

GARY COLEMAN: Maybe you'll never find your purpose.

CHRISTMAS EVE: Lots of people don't.

PRINCETON: But then, I don't know why I'm even alive!

KATE MONSTER: Well, who does, really? Everyone's a little bit unsatisfied.

BRIAN: Everyone goes 'round a little empty inside.

GARY COLEMAN: Take a breath. Look around,

BRIAN: Swallow your pride,

KATE MONSTER: For now...

BRIAN, KATE, GARY, CHRISTMAS EVE: For now...

NICKY: Nothing lasts,

ROD: Life goes on,

NICKY: Full of surprises.

ROD: You'll be faced with problems of all shapes and sizes.

CHRISTMAS EVE: You're going to have to make a few compromises... For now...

TREKKIE MONSTER: For now...

LUCY: For now we're healthy.

BRIAN: For now we're employed.

BAD IDEA BEARS: For now we're happy...

KATE MONSTER: If not overjoyed.

PRINCETON: And we'll accept the things we cannot avoid, for now...
Only for now! (For now there's life!)
Only for now! (For now there's love!)
Only for now! (For now there's work!)
For now there's happiness!
But only for now! (For now there's comfort!)
Only for now! (For now there's friendship!)
Only for now (For now!)
Only for now!
Only for now! (Sex!)
Is only for now! (Your hair!)
Is only for now! (George Bush!)
Is only for now!

Don't stress,
Relax,
Let life roll off your backs
Except for death and paying taxes,
Everything in life is only for now!

NICKY: Each time you smile...

ALL: ...Only for now

KATE MONSTER: It'll only last a while.

ALL: ...Only for now

PRINCETON: Life may be scary...

ALL: ...Only for now

But it's only temporary

PRINCETON: Everything in life is only for now.

Indeed, the perception of life is very important. When we reach a state of mind and spirit where we can look at things in the simplest way, we have attained a much higher plateau of spiritual development. We will be rid of emotional stress, perhaps our largest toxic health risk.

The following view of life will help you eliminate the unnecessary stress:

The PingLongevity™ State of Mind

- Without me, the earth will continue to turn. Everything is temporary, be it the president, the billionaires, the movie stars!

- Success depends on both fate and deeds! I'll do my best. But after that, it's up to the fate that only God controls. I am content and happy, accepting my fate. If it is not mine, no matter what I crave, it won't be mine.

- I don't judge others because each one came to the world destined to play a role, good or evil, beautiful or ugly, great or ordinary. Without the variety, the world does not exist.

- I don't have ego. I am content to lay low. Low does not have to be small. It can be vast and great, like the ocean where all rivers converge! That's true leadership in life.

- When my spirit leaves my physical body, I cannot take fame, power and money with me. But I can be a higher developed spirit than when I first arrived in this world.

- The seven emotions, overjoy, sadness, anger, overthinking, grief, fear and fright, cannot invade me. They are simply manifestations of fateful events. They are simply worldly.

- If you have to be the best, you'll always be bettered.

> "Dan, a very successful billionaire businessman, came to my office a few years ago. He was always on the phone, busy dealing with businesses all over the world. After he read our book *Asian Longevity Secrets,* he was drawn to Taoism. He searched and read more than ten books on Taoism. He completely changed his view of life and reduced his stress.
>
> 'Dr. Ping, you've changed my life,' he told me. 'Not only my health, but the way I think, the way I deal with people. I'm much happier and less stressed.'"
>
> —Dr. Ping

6.4.4   TCM Method for Emotional Wellbeing

In Sections 5.1 and 5.2, we discussed that your organ meridian systems influence your emotional wellbeing and vice versa. By unblocking your energy meridians and rebalancing your organs, you'll enjoy a focused clear mind, supported by positive emotions.

The liver system is very important to our emotional well-being. When the liver meridian is blocked and unbalanced, you become irritable and angry. You feel overwhelmed, unable to deal with all the tasks at hand. You become stressed and depressed easily.

We have great success with herbal formulas by detoxifying and tonicking the liver, for example, using Xiao Chai Hu Tang, Jia Wei

Xiao Yao, Gan Mai Da Zao, and Long Dan Xie Gan, all formulas that have been proven over thousands of years of use.

Other methods may include using acupuncture to do the same. We have seen so many clinical cases where patients come back to report that they feel "good," "grounded to the earth," "connected to surroundings." They changed their attitude towards people. They become cheerful and more social.

6.5   SUMMARY

This chapter offers the following points:

From the viewpoints of both modern science and TCM, emotional stress, greed and craving can be deadly to your body, mind and spirit. It's a major contributor to make you old fast. If you want vibrant health and longevity, you must become a better spiritual being.

There are several ways of releasing stress:

• Use chi-gong methods: Perform daily meditations for at least 30 minutes before bed. Make sure to achieve ultra-stillness and emptiness, which are more important than the length of time you meditate. Usually when you start, it may take a long time to reach this chi-gong state. After you practice for a while, you will be able to reach the chi-gong state immediately.

• Compartmentalize your time so that stressors are always confined within a set schedule.

• Adopt a Taoist view of the world. Try your best, and then accept the results as they are.

• Consider taking a liver tonic and detoxifying herbs.

Let's conclude by quoting the *Tao-De-Ching,* one of the world's most printed books, by Lao Tzu.

The five colors blind the eye,
The five tones deafen the ear,
The five flavors dull the taste,
Racing and hunting madden the mind,
Precious things lead one astray.

Therefore the sage is guided by what he feels
    and not by what he sees.
He lets go of that and chooses this.
Yield and overcome;
Bend and be straight;
Empty and be full;
Wear out and be new;
Have little and gain;
Have much and be confused.

Therefore wise men embrace the one
And set an example to all.
Not putting on a display,
They shine forth.
Not justifying themselves,
They are distinguished.
Not boasting,
They receive recognition.
Not bragging,
They never falter.
They do not quarrel,
So no one quarrels with them.

Therefore the ancients say, "Yield and overcome."
Is that an empty saying?
Be really whole,
And all things will come to you.

CHAPTER 7

Youthful Hormones
for Life

You may wonder why:

- No matter how you tried to diet, you still don't lose weight;

- No matter how many calcium supplements you take, you still get osteoporosis

- You are exposed to a higher risk of cardiovascular disease in middle age;

- Men get enlarged prostate and prostate cancer after middle age;

- Women get breast cancer and ovarian cancer in their middle age;

- You lose muscles and grow fat so easily in middle age;

- Men lose sexual virility and women lose sexual interest by middle age.

Hormone deterioration and imbalance are major root causes of all these problems. Hormones are our vital essence. If we lose vital essence, we are deprived of life force. Hormones are our control system. When they are out of whack, we lose control of our entire body system and disease is the result.

There are two primary control systems in our bodies, the nervous system, which sends electrical messages via neurons and the endocrine system using chemical messages via hormones. The endocrine system controls almost every cell, organ and function of our bodies. The endocrine system is instrumental in regulating mood, tissue function, metabolism, growth and development, as well as sexual function and reproductive processes.

Most endocrine hormones decline with age, creating imbalances. Hormonal imbalance is a fundamental cause of almost all degenerative diseases. Until recently, hormonal imbalance and the resulting symptoms and diseases have been viewed as the normal course of aging.

PingLongevity™ Hormone is a set of protocols to help you sustain youthful hormones for as long as possible through a safe and scientifically based system. Our goal is to delay drug intervention using natural methods for most of our lives, until we absolutely need them.

7.1   THE HORMONAL CONTROL SYSTEM

The endocrine system consists of hormones, which are chemical messengers, endocrine glands, which secrete hormones, hormone receptors that reside in every cell to receive control signals and the transport system through the blood vessels.

Our body's primary endocrine glands are: hypothalamus, pineal, pituitary, parathyroid, thyroid, thymus, adrenal, pancreas, ovary (female) and testis (male). See the figure on the following page for their locations.

A single gland or cell may secrete multiple hormones and multiple glands may secrete the same single hormone. The pituitary gland is called the "master gland." It is under the control of the hypothalamus. Together, their hormones control the hormone secretion of many other endocrine glands.

Hormones usually work in antagonistic pairs for checks and balances. For example, as we discussed in Section 6.2.1, adrenaline is the "fight, flight or freeze" hormone, acetylcholine the "rest and digest" hormone. Much hormonal regulation depends on negative feedback loops to maintain balance and homeostasis so the function that the hormones regulate is not too high or too low. Once the brain

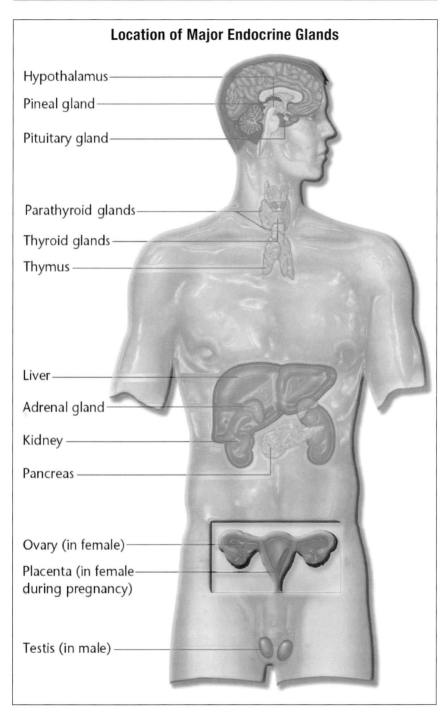

Location of Major Endocrine Glands

Hypothalamus

Pineal gland

Pituitary gland

Parathyroid glands

Thyroid glands

Thymus

Liver

Adrenal gland

Kidney

Pancreas

Ovary (in female)

Placenta (in female during pregnancy)

Testis (in male)

Courtesy of Dr. Bora Zivkovic, Scienceblogs.com.

knows there is an imbalance, it instructs one of these hormones to adjust the function up or down to regain balance.

Endocrine system disorder comes from:

- Hyposecretion due to secreting too little of a particular hormone,

- Hypersecretion due to secreting too much,

- Hyporesponsiveness due to a deficiency of receptors,

- Hyperresponsiveness due to overactive receptors.

As a result, the whole web of hormones becomes unbalanced.

Hormones secreted from the glands are transported through the bloodstream to all parts of the body, to specific targets.

Secretion of hormones may be controlled by neurons and other hormones through body's feedback loops.

Hormone receptors of various kinds reside in every cell. Hormones and receptors are like a key and lock. They must fit each other perfectly for the hormone to bind to the target cell in order to achieve the control effect. Hormone imbalance can occur due to either a lack of hormones or a malfunctioning or insensitive receptor function. For example, Type I diabetes is due to a lack of production of the hormone insulin by the pancreas. On the other hand, Type 2 diabetes results from insensitive receptors for insulin.

7.2   THE MAJOR HORMONAL AXES AND AGING

As we discussed in Section 1.2.2, our endocrine systems can become imbalanced in a dramatic way. Major decline and imbalance of hormones can occur along several major hormonal axes.

7.2.1   Growth and Repair

The growth hormone axis (GH axis) stimulates growth, cell reproduction and regeneration, stimulates the growth of bone and other body tissues and plays a role in the body's handling of nutrients and minerals. It is secreted by the pituitary gland. Since growth hormone levels fluctuate greatly throughout the day, IGF-1, insulin-like growth factor 1, is used as a screening test for growth hormone.

As you age, the growth hormone axis enters somatopause:

- Growth hormone decreases by 80% from the 20s to 60s;

- The ratio IGF-1/Insulin decreases dramatically, which many studies suggest is a cause of obesity and decreased lifespan.

- Deficiency in this axis may directly cause lost muscle, sagging skin, obesity and slow recovery and healing.

7.2.2 Metabolism Regulation

The hypothalamic-pituitary-thyroid axis (HPT axis) regulates metabolism, including body temperature and weight. Thyroid hormone Thyroxine (T4) is secreted by the thyroid gland. T4 is 99.95% bound by special type of proteins making it less active. T4 can be converted into the most active form of thyroid hormone triiodothyronine (T3). It can also be converted to the reverse T3 (rT3), which has the function of blocking the effect of thyroid hormone functions. The hypothalamus senses low circulating levels of thyroid hormone and responds by stimulating the pituitary to produce thyroid stimulating hormone (TSH). The TSH, in turn, stimulates the thyroid gland to produce more thyroid hormone until the feedback loop senses the level has become normal.

As you age, hypothalamic-pituitary-thyroid axis enters thyropause and potentially hypothyroidism:

- Total thyroid hormones decline with age;

- T3/T4 ratio dramatically reduces with age;

- T3/rT3 ratio dramatically reduced with age.

- Age related thyroid issues are: depression, memory loss, cognitive impairment and a variety of neuromuscular complaints.

7.2.3   Stress Regulation

The hypothalamic-pituitary-adrenal axis (HPA axis) regulates stress response. Feedback of environmental stressful stimuli initiates the hypothalamus to stimulate the release of the hormone adrenocorticotrophic hormone, which in turn instructs the adrenal glands to release cortisol. Cortisol affects the body's reaction to stress, as we discussed in Section 6.2.1, among other functions such as regulation of salt and water balance, until the feedback loop senses the level has reached where it needs to be.

The hypothalamic-pituitary-adrenal axis enters adrenopause, or adrenal fatique:

- DHEA declines from the 20s to the 60s by 74% in men, and 64% in women;

- The stress hormone, cortisol tends to increase first, then decline with age;

- DHEA/cortisol ratio significantly decreases with age;

- Adrenopause causes a decline of immune response and increase in diabetes, atherosclerosis, dementia, obesity and osteoporosis.

7.2.4   Glucose Control

The pancreas produces, among other things, two primary hormones: insulin and glucagon. They work together to maintain a steady level of glucose or sugar, in the blood. Insulin and glucagon have opposite effects on the liver's control of blood sugar level. Insulin lowers the blood sugar level by instructing the liver to take glucose out of circulation and store it, while glucagon instructs the liver to release some of its stored supply to raise the blood sugar level.

In the insulin axis, metabolic syndrome tends to develop as we age:

- Blood serum glucose rises;

- Insulin resistance (Type 2 diabetes) due to insensitive insulin receptors becomes prevalent.

- Diseases related to metabolic syndrome are: high blood pressure, high cholesterol, high triglycerides, high blood sugar, high insulin levels and obesity.

7.2.5   Sex, Reproduction and Aging

The hypothalamic-pituitary-gonadal axis (HPG axis) controls the development and regulation of development, reproduction, immune systems and aging. Like other feedback loops, the hypothalamus senses insufficiencies and instructs the pituitary to produce luteinizing hormone (LH) and follicle-stimulating hormone (FSH), which in turn regulate the release of sex hormones.

In men, the testes secrete hormones called androgens, including testosterone. Testosterone can either directly act upon receptors, or convert to dihydrotestosterone (DHT), a more potent version of testosterone, by the enzyme 5-alpha reductase and to estradiol, a version of female sex hormone, by the enzyme aromatase.

Approximately 5% of serum testosterone produced in men undergoes 5α-reduction to form DHT. DHT has three times greater affinity for androgen receptors than testosterone, meaning it's much more potent. During embryogenesis, DHT has an essential role in the formation of the male external genitalia. Studies show that DHT has a negative role in causing hair loss and prostate cancer in adult male when the ratio testosterone/DHT decreases.

Liver has a significant role in metabolizing hormones. For example, excess estrogens in the blood are eliminated by the liver. An impaired or stagnated liver is a root cause of hormone imbalance. If the liver is malfunctioning, male estrogen dominance may arise.

Most testosterone in the blood is bound by sex hormone-binding globulin (SHBG), making it inactive. Therefore, it's important to measure the bio-available and free testosterone.

Testosterone is critical for fetal development, secondary male sex characteristics, sperm production, libido, healing, muscle development, fat burning and many other functions.

Men begin andropause in their late 40s or as early as mid 30s with gradual hormonal changes:

- Testosterone declines by approximately 7% and free testosterone by 14% every decade after peaking at the ages of 18 to 22;

- Testosterone/estrogen ratio decreases by 12% per decade, thus becoming "estrogen dominant;"

- Testosterone/DHT ratio declines significantly with age;

- Sexual vitality reduces significantly. Between the ages of 20 and 60, frequency of sexual orgasms reduces by about 65% from about 104 times a year to 35 times, and erection angle for men declines from 20 degrees to –25 degrees;

- The liver become congested, impairing the inactivation and elimination of excess estrogens.

- An imbalance in the hypothalamic-pituitary-gonadal axis for men has been shown to have widespread impact on the body such as erectile dysfunction, loss of libido, depression, lack of energy, loss of muscle size and strength, osteoporosis, heart disease, increased body fat, Type 2 diabetes, obesity, prostate cancer, Alzheimer's and insomnia, just to name a few.

> "Men with low testosterone had a 33% greater death risk over their next 18 years of life compared with men who had higher testosterone, according to the study conducted by Dr. Elizabeth Barrett-Connor and colleagues at the University of California at San Diego."
> —*ABC NEWS*, JUNE 6, 2007

The female gonads, the ovaries, are located in the pelvis. They produce eggs and secrete the hormones estrogen and progesterone. They also secrete the male hormone testosterone, which is an important part of female physiology. In addition to the ovary, the adrenal glands also secrete a relatively small quantity of estrogen and testosterone and fat tissues produce some estrogen as well.

Estrogen is involved in the development of female sexual features such as breast growth, the accumulation of body fat around the hips and thighs and the growth spurt that occurs during puberty.

The pair, estrogen and progesterone, together regulate pregnancy and the menstrual cycle.

There are three major types of estrogen: estrone (E1), estradiol (E2), and estriol (E3). Estradiol (E2) is the predominant form in non-pregnant women and is nearly nonexistent by the time a woman reaches menopause, estrone is produced during menopause, and estriol is the primary estrogen in pregnancy. E1 may further convert to two metabolites, 2-hydroxyestrone (2-OH-E1) and 16-Alpha-hydroxyestrone (16-a-OH-E1), the ratio of which is a very important predictor of cancer. The 16 form is much more potent than the 2 form. As we age, the ratio changes, causing degenerative diseases such as cancer.

In a normal adult woman, estrogen rises from the lowest at the start of the 28-day menstrual cycle (initial heavy flow of menstruation) to its highest peak at ovulation on day 14, reaching a second peak on day 21, then continuing its decline until day 28, when the menstrual period begins. Progesterone is produced immediately after ovulation (day 14) to prepare the uterus for reception and development of the fertilized egg. The level peaks at day 21. If no fertilization takes place, it gradually falls back to very low level towards day 28. If pregnancy occurs, both estrogen and progesterone increase and maintain at high level to promote the development of the fetus.

At the onset of puberty around ages 10–15, estradiol gradually increases to about 20–40% of that of a mature woman of age 15 and older, while progesterone increases to 37–50% of that of a mature woman.

During perimenopause, menopause and postmenopause, estradiol and progesterone continue to fall to a level as low as 5% and 3%, respectively of that of a young adult level.

Women usually begin *menopause* in their late 40s and perimenopause as early as mid 30s. At menopause,

• Estrogen declines by 35%;

• Progesterone declines by 75%;

- Progesterone/Estrogen ratio decreases by 38%, becoming "estrogen dominant;"

- E2/E1 ratio decreases dramatically;

- 2-hydroxyestrone/16-hydroxyestrone ratio dramatic decreases.

- An imbalance in this axis for women has been shown to have a widespread impact on the body. It's been linked to autoimmune diseases (rheumatoid arthritis and psoriasis), cardiovascular diseases, osteoporosis, breast and ovarian cancer, loss of libido, depression, lack of energy, loss of muscle size and strength, increased body fat, Type 2 diabetes, obesity, Alzheimer's and insomnia, just to name a few.

7.2.6   Other Hormonal Axis

There are many other hormones for other body functions. For example, parathyroid hormone, secreted by the parathyroid glands, regulates the level of calcium in the blood and is important to prevent osteoporosis; prolactin by pituitary gland for milk production in women and sexual gratification in the refractory period for both sexes; melatonin by the pineal gland for regulation of sleep and wake cycle and dehydrepiandrosterone (DHEA), an endogenous precursor hormone to male and female sex hormones (androgens and estrogens) produced by the adrenal glands.

7.3   THE RISKS OF HORMONE THERAPIES

As discussed in Section 7.2, a hormone system imbalance can result in many severe degenerative diseases. Thus keeping a youthful hormone level and balance is of fundamental importance to vibrant health and longevity! However, as important as it is, there's also a high risk associated with tinkering with our hormone systems. It is the most complex control system in our bodies. Tuned improperly, hormone imbalance can cause serious diseases.

   Most of us have experienced car trouble. You see a warning light about your ignition system. You take the car to your mechanic, who checks and checks, replaces several parts in the fuel control system, costing you a bunch of money. The warning light stays on. He tries something else, change more parts, tunes up more controls, charging you more service fees. After all is done, the car is still not fixed. You start all over again with another shop and then another, trying to figure out the problem.

Your hormone system is much the same, but infinitely more complex. It is a similar dilemma: You don't want someone who doesn't know what he or she is doing tinkering with your hormonal system without success. In fact, the risk is extremely high if you are dealing with someone who doesn't know how to fine tune the hormonal system.

This section will talk about some of the intricacies and risks in artificially modulated hormones. It's not designed to scare you away. We are simply trying to educate you about the risk so you'll know more about potential treatments if you need them.

7.3.1   Hormone Pathway Complexity

The endocrine system is a very complex web. Hormones are interrelated, and many times, under certain enzymatic actions, they can convert to one another. Take, for example, steroid hormones, the group of hormones produced through cholesterol. The graph on the following page shows the complex interrelationship.

"I have seen patients who came in with testosterone replacement at other clinics due to low testosterone and impotence, weight gain, muscle loss and lack of energy. Upon looking at their previous lab results, I found that their doctors only monitored testosterone and free testosterone. No other hormones were measured. I wondered how the doctors could possibly know what's going on without testing an entire spectrum of hormones. For example, testosterone can be converted into estradiol and DHT. How does the doctor really know his replacement hormones went through the correct pathway? How does he steer the pathway with the correct treatment plan? I've heard doctor friends talking about body builders using steroids in hopes of getting bigger muscles, only to grow breasts instead."

—DR. PING WU

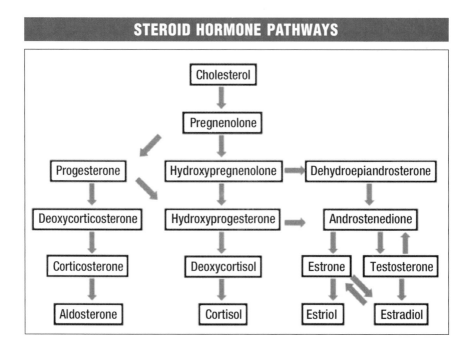

STEROID HORMONE PATHWAYS

7.3.2   Hormones Are a Complex Interconnected Web

Since hormones are interrelated, sometimes problems in one pathway, for example, testosterone deficiency, may be caused by issues in other axes, such as thyroid issues.

An example given by Dr. Eugene Shippen demonstrates how interrelated these pathways are. As a man ages, his body tends to try to keep his estradiol level as constant as possible, probably due to the importance of the hormone in a male body. The body does this by converting the already declining testosterone to estradiol. A high estradiol level then further depresses the pituitary hormones LH and FSH, which in turn lowers the production of testosterone (Section 7.2.5). Reduced testosterone also depresses the release of growth hormones. The net effect then causes insulin resistance (Section 7.2.4), which increases body fat. Since body fat is loaded with estradiol and the testosterone-estradiol conversion enzyme aromatase, it further helps the production of estradiol (Section 7.2.5). In the meantime, fat cells also increase inflammation cytokine, which causes stress and increases cortisol while decreasing DHEA (Section 7.2.3). Cortisol suppresses the production of thyroid hormone T3, and increases of rT3 (Section 7.2.2). This results in an increase of the hormone prolactin (Section 7.2.6), which further increases E2 conversion and reduces testosterone production.

As you may see, the hormone pathways are interrelated. As in the above example, you may experience symptoms of multiple dysfunctions of axes. You may have andropause, or thyropause, or adrenopause, or metabolic syndrome or more than one of the previous conditions. Where to start? Which one is the root cause of this cascade of problems?

7.3.3 Difficulty in Setting Target Levels

As we discussed in Section 1.4.1, there's a large range of medical "normal." For example, suppose that a man is tested with, in the example of Section 1.4.1, a testosterone level of 500 ng/dL against a "normal" level of 270–1070 ng/dL, is he high or low?

The combination, or the balance of hormones, is even more telling. Suppose furthermore he is tested with estradiol of 40 pg/mL against normal of 21–50, DHT of 45 ng/dL against 15–55, SHBG of 63 nmol/L against 13–71, free testosterone of 1%, is he normal? What should be the correct ratios among these hormones in order to achieve the balance that is optimal to you as an individual, rather than a statistical average? Now you get the point. It can be a vast ocean where the doctors need to pick up a point of reference to move your hormones toward.

7.3.4 Drug Dependency

As discussed in Section 7.1.2, the body keeps hormone levels balanced through a feedback loop. Most of the feedback is managed by the hypothalamus, which senses the lack of or sufficiency of particular hormones in the blood stream. It issues commands to slow or speed hormone production.

When we add external hormones into our systems, we basically tell the brain that we have an increase of these particular hormones. The brain will then reduce or shut down the body's internal production. Over time, our internal glands may lose their ability to produce that hormone. For example, some people using testosterone replacement therapy experience shrinking testicles.

Usually, once external hormones are added to the body, the body learns to be dependent on them. Therefore, unless you really need hormone replacement, it is best to first determine if you can get your own body to function through natural means.

7.3.5   Uncertain Long-Term Impact

The Women's Health Initiative (WHI) was launched in 1991 and consisted of a set of clinical trials and an observational study, which together involved 161,808 generally healthy postmenopausal women. In its estrogen plus progestin (a synthetic progesterone drug) hormone replacement trial, the WHI concluded with the risks.

- **Breast cancer:** The risk of developing breast cancer in women not taking HRT (on placebo) was 30 per 10,000 women-years. On HRT, the risk was 38 per 10,000 women-years.

- **Heart disease:** Women not taking HRT had 30 cases of heart disease per 10,000 women-years. Women on HRT had 37 cases per 10,000 women-years.

- **Stroke:** On a placebo, the risk was 21 per 10,000. On HRT, the risk was 29 per 10,000.

- **Clots in the veins (venous thrombosis):** On a placebo, the risk was 16 per 10,000. On HRT, the risk was 34 per 10,000. Researchers included those clots that moved from the leg veins up into the lungs, which are the most dangerous type, as well as those that stayed within the leg veins.

- **Endometrial cancer:** It is difficult to put an exact figure on this, but long-term estrogen-only HRT does increase the risk of abnormal growth of the lining of the womb (endometrium) and endometrial cancer. Using combined HRT reduces, but does not eliminate, the risk. Evidence suggests that sequential combined HRT may still be associated with slightly increased risk of endometrial cancer, however no increased risk has been found with continuous combined HRT.

Many experts argue that synthetic hormones are the underlying cause of these side effects. However, we believe most likely it is due to incorrect treatment protocols, due to reasons discussed in Sections 7.3.1–7.3.4. Of course, no one wants to be reassured by a doctor that a medication is safe, only to find out about its dangerous side effects decades later!

7.4 HORMONE BALANCING AND REPLACEMENT THERAPIES

For a long life, we must keep our hormones from becoming unbalanced or declining for as long as possible. This is the ultimate fountain of youth. At the same time, we want to avoid the pitfalls and risks of hormone therapies discussed in Section 7.3.

PingLongevity™ Hormone therapy is based on the following principles:

7.4.1 Step 1: Baseline Your Optimal Hormone Level

As discussed in Section 1.4.1, your body's optimal condition is set around age 18 to 22. However, between ages 22 and 35, most of us are reasonably healthy. You should do a thorough baseline of all health parameters as early as you can. If you have done this, you're among the very lucky ones. This is because no one really knows your optimal level. Each one of us is genetically so unique, and the variation among us is huge. That's why the "normal" range is so large.

If you've already experienced declining health and unbalanced hormones and have yet to be able to do a baseline, you'll have to go through some trial and error. Start with a comprehensive Ping-Longevity™ Test, including the hormone profile test. From these tests, you can start treatment using tiny incremental steps, until your follow-up laboratory tests and hormone profile tests show improvement.

In retaining current hormone levels or restoring primary hormones towards the baseline, it's critically important that we target not only the absolute hormone levels, but also the following ratios:

- IGF-1/Insulin;

- T3/T4 and T3/rT3;

- DHEA/cortisol;

- Testosterone/estradiol (male);

- Testosterone/DHT (male);

- Progesterone/estrogen (female);

- E2/E1 (female);

- 2-hydroxyestrone/16-hydroxyestrone (female)

One exception to the 18- to 22-year-old optimal baseline rule is for the sex hormones of perimenopausal and menopausal women. If you restore hormones to those of an 18- to 22-year-old, you'll restore your menstrual periods, which may not be necessary or desirable. Therefore, there may be several options:

- Use your 18- to 22-year-old hormones as the baseline. Some hormone doctors believe that even for menopausal women, it's good to supplement hormones in a similar dosage and timing to reinitiate monthly menstruation. PingLongevity™ Hormone recommends a lighter hormone supplementation therapy.

- Use a lighter therapy to eliminate all or a majority symptoms in the female hormone profile test (Section 1.4.4), while at the same time referencing the relative ratios from your 18 to 22 baseline. This usually means to balance all the ratios to your optimal level without restoring the absolute level all the way. For most menopausal women, this is what PingLongevity™ Hormone recommends.

- Mimic the hormones at pregnancy. There have been studies showing that pregnancy has a beneficial effect on women and can reduce cancer rates and extend life. The beneficial effects of progesterone, and the hormone estriol (E3), which are high during pregnancy, are generally credited for the hormone's positive effects. Thus, to mimic pregnancy hormones, we might create a balanced preparation of 25% estradiol, 25% estrone, and 50% estriol, plus progesterone. The quantity and timing is based on a qualitative test of daily and monthly estrogen dominance or deficiency.

- Based on a protocol first proposed by Dr. Taichi Tzu and Dr. Ping Wu in 2001, this option is based on the following hypothesis:

  The Least Women's Vital Essence Consumption Hypothesis: The most life preserving sex hormone level for a women, optimizing healthy life span and maximum life span is similar to those of her Tanner Stage III, regardless of her adult age.

In Taoist alchemy, as will be discussed in Section 7.5, it is believed that a woman's optimal sex hormone baseline should be the ones when she was in her early teens, prior to the onset of puberty. This usually means estradiol, estriol and progesterone levels to be near or less than one-half of those of when you were a young adult (age 15–22). One of the ultimate goals of Taoist alchemy is to train the body, while still young, healthy and vital, to stop menstruation and restore it to its pre-puberty state. It is said, in ancient Taoist literature, that once this is achieved, a woman's breasts are like those of a pre-pubertal teen. The process of stopping menstruation in Taoist alchemy is called the "chopped red dragon," referring to the stoppage of menstrual blood. This will be more extensively discussed in Section 7.4.3.

Although this may be an optimal and beneficial target for women, it is probably the most advanced and most unrealistic one if you want to live a normal life. For example, once you restore hormones to pre-puberty levels, childbirth is out of the question. Without supervision and an advanced Taoist master's face-to-face teaching, we do not recommend this target.

Another exception to the 18 to 22 rule is that, for middle-aged men, it is not necessary to restore or maintain the same level of DHT. This is because DHT has lost some its main function and may become a liability in adult males.

Once we set the baseline, it'll be a goal to move the body towards the optimal. However, many patients will experience dramatic health benefits even without completely restoring them to the baseline. Therefore, return to baseline is the goal, not necessarily the end result.

7.4.2   Step 2: Lifestyle Hormone Optimization

The best way to have youthful hormone levels is not to let hormones get old in the first place. In previous chapters, we talked about many ways of maintaining youthful hormones. In particular:

- The PingLongevity™ Diet will maintain the best insulin-glucose axis because it never spikes insulin, so the body becomes very insulin sensitive, as discussed in Sections 2.2.2 and 7.2.4.

- Our detoxification protocols help eliminate the toxins such as alcohol and chemical drugs, which studies have shown to lower major hormones, as discussed in Section 2.10.1.

- PingLongevity™ Caloric Restriction can help dramatically delay the onset of aging and maintain hormones at youthful levels for much longer than usual, benefitting all the hormonal axes, as discussed in Section 3.3.6;

- Avoid farmed fish, chicken and beef because they frequently contain artificially fed hormones, which impact your hormone balance.

- Avoid using chemical products such as deodorants, perfumes, shampoos and conditioners. Recently, a pediatrician from Massachusetts found that many pre-teen and teenage boys come to see him with enlarged breasts. After taking a careful case history, he pinpointed the root cause: The boys were using a very popular name brand shampoo and bubble bath. He further confirmed that one of the ingredients is indeed associated with breast enlargement. So now we recommend you to use natural soap and oils, personal care products and cosmetics.

- Avoid excessive use of alcohol and recreational drugs. Many teenagers are having erectile problems due to liver damage due to using drugs and drinking alcoholic beverages, which decrease sex hormones.

> "Janet, a 50-year-old, with heavy menopause symptoms that included night sweats soaking her night gown and severe hot flashes every 20 minutes in the day time. After detoxifying her liver, rebalancing her hormones, cooling her system and nourishing her yin energy, all her symptoms were gone. Her period even came back naturally after it had stopped for a full year. She tells me that now, if she drinks wine at dinner, she'll have night sweats for the next couple of nights."
>
> —Dr. Ping

7.4.3   Step 3: Taoist Alchemy

We'll discuss Taoist alchemy in section 7.5 This very effective ancient method from the sages of Taoism, transforms sexual energy, can help dramatically delay the aging of hormonal systems. It's a natural method, requiring no drugs or even particular foods and yet has tremendous impact on all steroid hormones. Taoist alchemy provides an effective means of stimulating hormone production, activating receptors in the entire body and preserving vital hormonal essence and energy.

7.4.4   Step 4: Food Hormone Therapy

There are classes of foods known to impact various types of hormones. This will be covered in Section 7.6.

7.4.5   Step 5: Natural Hormone Balancing

By using certain herbs and supplements, we can effectively inhibit 5a-reductase to prevent the conversion of testosterone to DHT, inhibit aromatase to minimize testosterone conversion to estradiol, enhance liver detoxification to eliminate excess estrogen and increase hormone production (Section 7.2.5). This will be discussed in Section 7.7.

7.4.6   Step 6: Bio-identical Hormone Therapy

When all the methods in Steps 2 through 5 still do not yield an optimal hormone level, drug intervention may be required. Bio-identical hormone therapy is believed to be much safer and more beneficial than synthetic hormone therapy. This will be covered in chapter 9 as an intervention method.

7.5   TAOIST ALCHEMY FOR TRANSFORMING VITAL ENERGY

Sexual energy and sex hormones represent our virility and vitality, from the points of view of the thousands of years of Traditional Chinese Medicine as well as modern sciences. This sexual energy and its accompanying hormones are our life force and vital essence, without which we become old.

Taoist alchemy has a unique way of preserving this vital essence so that we can sustain youthful hormones for longer, transforming sexual energy into higher spiritual energy to benefit all aspects of life.

7.5.1   Sexual Energy as the Life Force

Life force, chi, energy, vitality—all are terms for a collection of life-sustaining prenatal and postnatal substances (hormones, blood, etc.) and higher energies (Chapter 10), which science has yet to fully measure and comprehend.

Sexual energy is considered the most important and powerful life force by both Traditional Chinese Medicine and modern science. It defines our lives, longevity and life force.

In the ancient book, *Yellow Emperor's Classics of Internal Medicine* there is the following dialog:

"Yellow Emperor: When a man grows old, he cannot have children. Is it because his energy has already been exhausted or because it is a natural phenomenon?

Chi-Po replied: The kidney energy of a woman becomes abundant at the age of 7, her baby teeth begin to be replaced by permanent ones and her hair begins to grow longer. At the age of 14, a woman will begin to menstruate. Her conception meridian begins to flow and the energy in her connective meridian begins to grow in abundance and she begins to menstruate and she is capable of becoming pregnant. At the age of 21, the kidney energy of a woman becomes equal to an average adult and for that reason; her last tooth begins to grow with all other teeth completed.

At the age of 28, tendons and bones become hard, the hair grows to its greatest length and her body is in the top condition. At the age of 35, the bright Yang meridians begin to weaken with the result that her complexion starts to look withered and her hair begins to fall out. At the age of 42, the three Yang meridians begin to weaken with the result that her complexion starts to look even more withered and her hair begins to turn gray. At the age of 49, the energy of the conception meridian becomes deficient, the energy of the connective meridian becomes weakened and scanty, the sexual energy becomes exhausted and menstruation stops with the result that her body becomes old and she cannot become pregnant any longer.

For a man, his kidney energy becomes abundant, his hair begins to grow longer, and his teeth begin to change at the age of 8. At the age of 16, his kidney energy becomes even more abundant, his sexual energy begins to arrive, he is full of semen that he can ejaculate. When he has sexual intercourse with woman, he can have children.

At the age of 24, the kidney energy of a man becomes equal to an average adult with strong tendons and bones; his last tooth begins to grow with all other teeth are completed. At the age of 32, all tendons, bones and muscles are already fully grown. At the age of 40, the kidney energy begins to weaken, hair begins to fall out and teeth begin to wither. At the age of 48, a weakening and exhaustion of Yang energy begins to take place in upper region, with the result that his complexion begins to look withered and his hair begins to turn gray.

At the age of 56, the liver energy begins to weaken, the tendons become inactive, the sexual energy begins to dissipate, the semen becomes scanty, the kidneys become weakened with the result that all parts of the body begin to grow old. At the age 64, hair and teeth are gone.

The kidneys are in charge of water, and they receive pure energy from the five viscera and the six bowels and store it. For this reason, it is only when the five viscera are full of energy that ejaculation is possible. Now the five viscera have already wakened, the tendons and bones have already become relaxed and powerless, it is quite natural that the sexual energy is also exhausted. This is the reason that hair on the head and at the temples turns gray, that the body becomes heavy and his steps become inaccurate and that he cannot have children any longer.

It is necessary to know about menstruation in women and growth of sex energy in men; without such knowledge, one is bound to grow old early."

—*YELLOW EMPEROR'S CLASSICS OF INTERNAL MEDICINE*

In traditional Chinese medicine, kidney meridian, kidney energy and sexual energy are all related to the system of hormonal glands, including the adrenals, testes and ovaries and the hormones that include growth hormones, DHEA, testosterone, estrogen, and progesterone.

The procreation theory is one of the theories of aging that are espoused by modern science as discussed in Section 1.3.1. The theory includes the concept that the procreation of the next generation of human beings is the priority purpose of our existence. Once that task is achieved, we are on a declining path that ultimately leads to death. Those who experience early puberty, according to this theory, have an early start in consuming their reproductive reservoirs and expending their sexual energy and as a result, they will become old and die at an earlier age.

Scientists divide human life into three main stages: childhood (from birth to puberty), adulthood (reproductive years) and senescence (post reproduction).

The first stage is also called the entropy stage. This is because the human body possesses the property of negative entropy, i.e., it is continuously seeking a state of increased organization. The second stage is called the plateau phase. In this phase, we gradually release energy (limited potential) to sustain life, so life is gradually washed away. The third stage is the rapid descent phase, in which life quickly degenerates—the maximum rate of entropy toward *dis*organization.

It is also interesting to note that the "ability to reproduce" (puberty) signals the start of the decline of life. Somehow, the activity of reproduction (or sex) has to pay a price, a price of burning our life candles at a more rapid rate, reducing our health and longevity.

There seem to be extreme cases in nature that amplify this observation. For example, certain worms, fruit flies and Pacific salmon all die immediately after they reproduce. It seems that the purpose of their life is to reproduce. After that, they become useless and their deaths relieve a burden on their species. Others species die gradually after reproductive activities. This is true for most mammals.

In modern society, we have accelerated nature's course in the leaking of our vital essence. Most important, overnutrition has speeded up the onset of puberty.

"According to a study published this month in the journal *Pediatrics*, most white girls show signs of puberty before the age of 10, compared with about 15 at the turn of the 20th century."
—*NEWSWEEK MAGAZINE*, OCTOBER 18, 1999

7.5.2 Health Benefit of Sexual Activities

Many scientific studies show that sexual activities are good for health. They dramatically stimulate sex hormone production and thus result in many health benefits.

In the insightful study titled, "Age and Seasonal Variation in Serum Testosterone Concentration among Men," published in 1990, Dr. J.M. Dabbs showed that successful love matches can cause testosterone to rise in both partners. Saliva testosterone concentration was measured in male and female members of four heterosexual couples on a total of 11 evenings before and after sexual intercourse and 11 evenings on which there was no intercourse. Testosterone increased during the evening when there was intercourse and decreased when there was none. The pattern was the same for males and females.

A January 7, 2010 report on *CNN*, entitled, "New Year's Resolution, Have More Sex," stated the following 10 benefits of regular sexual activity:

1. **A longer life:** In a British study, men who had intercourse at least twice a week lived longer than men who had sex less than once a month. A U.S. study had similar findings and a Swedish study examining the sex lives of 70-year-olds found that men who died before their 75th birthdays had ceased having sexual intercourse at earlier ages. The Swedish study didn't find that women lived longer if they had sex more frequently and neither did a study in North Carolina. However, in the North Carolina study, women who reported enjoying sex more often lived longer than those who didn't report enjoyment.

2. **A healthier heart:** In a British study, people who had intercourse twice a week or more were less likely to have heart

attacks and other fatal coronary events. Those who had sex less than once a month had twice the rate of fatal coronary events, compared with those with the highest frequency of intercourse.

3. **Lower blood pressure:** In a study published in the journal *Biological Psychology*, people who had sex more often tended to have lower diastolic blood pressure, or the bottom number in a blood pressure reading. Brody's experiment, in which more sexually active study subjects had markedly fewer dramatic blood pressure spikes when they were put under stress, also supports the benefit.

4. **Lower risk of breast cancer:** A French study found that women who have vaginal intercourse not at all or infrequently had three times the risk of breast cancer, compared with women who had intercourse more often.

5. **Lower risk of prostate cancer:** A Minnesota study found that men who'd had intercourse more than 3,000 times in their lives had half the prostate cancer risk of those who had not. While it's not clear why this would be true, studies have found that men who had more intercourse tended to have better prostate function and eliminated more waste products in their semen. "These differences could conceivably impact prostate cancer risk," Brody writes in his article.

6. **Pain relief:** Whipple and others have conducted studies suggesting that more sexual activity helps relieve lower back pain and migraines.

7. **A slimmer physique:** A study of healthy German adults revealed that men and women who had sex more frequently tended to be slimmer than folks who didn't have as much sex. Sex burns 50 to 60 calories per encounter, Whipple says, so sex three times a week for a month would burn about 700 calories—or the equivalent of jogging about seven miles.

8. **Better testosterone levels:** A group of men being treated for erectile problems saw greater increases in testosterone when,

along with the treatments, they had frequent sex. Specifically, men who had sex at least eight times per month had greater increases than those who had sex less than eight times per month.

9. **Fewer menopause symptoms:** Menopausal women in Nigeria experienced fewer hot flashes when they had sex more frequently. Brody says this may be because sexual activity helps regulate hormonal levels, which in turn affect the symptoms of menopause.

10. **Healthier semen:** In three studies, men who had frequent intercourse had a higher volume of semen, a higher sperm count and a higher percentage of healthier sperm, compared with men who tended to participate in other sexual activities."

7.5.3   The Depletion of Life Force

Indeed, if the start of puberty is the beginning of decline of life force, how is life force depleted?

In Taoist alchemy, it is believed that the way life force or sexual energy is depleted is different for men and women.

In men, life force is leaked due to orgasm with ejaculation of semen during sexual activities. Ancient sages believed that one drop of semen equaled one hundred drops of blood. The leakage consumes the body's most precious prenatal and postnatal vital essence.

Sex to men is a double-edged sword. On one hand, as discussed in Section 7.5.2, it stimulates all the body's production of testosterone, enhances the receptor capability, thus sustaining a more youthful hormone level. On the other hand, long-term frequent leakage of sexual energy (orgasm with ejaculation) can deplete life force, as discussed in Section 7.5.1. This is proven by modern sciences, despite its relative obscurity.

In the Chinese classic *Secret of the Jade Bedroom*, there is a dialog between the Yellow Emperor's two counselors, held 5,000 years ago:

"Rainbow girl: It is generally assumed that a man gains great pleasure from ejaculation. But when he learns the Tao of yin and yang, he will ejaculate less and less. Will this not diminish his pleasure as well?

Peng Tze: Not at all! After ejaculation, a man feels tired, his ears buzz, his eyes get heavy and he longs for sleep. He is thirsty and his limbs feel weak and stiff. By ejaculating, he enjoys a brief moment of sensation, but suffers long hours of weariness as a result. This is no true pleasure!

However, if a man regulates his ejaculation to an absolute minimum and retains his semen, his body will grow strong, his mind will be clear and his vision and hearing will improve. Is pre-serving sexual energy meant to reduce sexual pleasure?"

—SECRET OF THE JADE BEDROOM

Orgasm with ejaculation is regarded as the ultimate goal of recreational sex. Unfortunately, in addition to exciting peaks, orgasms produce powerful negative side-effects.

Ejaculation signals the body to produce more sperm. But the production of sperm signals the "age clock" to tick, accelerating the aging process. If you think back to the aging theory of reproduction, once the reproductive duty is performed, nature views the man to be useless, so he is supposed to deteriorate and die.

Two major hormones involved in sexual activities are dopamine, the reward hormone and prolactin, the hormone of satiation. When we become sexually excited, dopamine levels rise, reaching their peak at the time of orgasm. Some researchers compare this to the effects of heroin on the brain. After orgasm, dopamine levels fall sharply, accompanied by symptoms that mimic heroin withdrawal. At the same time, prolactin levels rise.

Prolactin signals the start of the post-orgasm hangover. These changes may last for days, corresponding to a lack of sexual urges.

If you think about it, many people experience tiredness after frequent sexual encounters. We tend to catch cold easily and want some rest. Some people even use sex as a kind of "sleeping pill."

"Like Balzac, who believed that a night of sex meant the loss of
a good page of his novel, so I believed that it meant the loss of
a good day's work at the studio."
        —CHARLIE CHAPLIN

According to a number of studies, many post-pubescent young
men report daily ejaculation and sometimes ejaculations several
times a day. When they reach their 40s, most men see this frequency
gradually decline to 2 or 3 times per week.

Thus, our sexual energy is overtaxed in modern society, typified
by earlier puberty and more expenditure of sexual energy, leading
to accelerated aging and the onset of degenerative diseases.

In women, Taoist Alchemy attributes the loss of life force to the
shedding of blood during menstruation. It is the process of menstruation, not necessarily the blood by itself, which leaks out a
woman's vital prenatal and postnatal essence and chi.

During ovulation, the associated hormones stimulate prenatal
and postnatal energies. The ovaries function under the control of
the pituitary gland, producing a hormone that stimulates follicle
growth and egg production, at the same time bringing about secretion of the hormone estrogen. This estrogen thickens the lining of
the uterus in preparation for receiving a fertilized egg. Then the
hormone progesterone is produced. If the egg is not fertilized, progesterone production is halted and the lining of the uterus is shed
during the monthly menstrual period. Thus the cycle starts again
for the next month.

Taoists believe that this reproductive cycle requires significant
energy expenditure, just as the release of semen does in men.

During menstruation, a woman may feel the loss of life force.
She may feel tired, short- tempered, bloated, moody and listless.

Indeed, there's some modern support of this viewpoint. A
woman is born with a limited number of eggs; one to two million
immature eggs or follicles are stored in the ovaries. When she
reaches puberty and starts to menstruate, only about 400,000 follicles remain. With each menstrual cycle, a thousand follicles are lost
and only one lucky one will actually mature into an ovum (egg),

which is released into the fallopian tube at the onset of ovulation.

That means that of the one to two million follicles with which she is born, only about 400 will mature in the entire life of a woman. When a woman reaches menopause, she has essentially no follicles left.

The process of menstruation is like a life clock that deducts your vitality potential one month at a time.

7.5.4   The Framework of Taoist Internal Alchemy

In describing Taoist internal alchemy, we'll try to use the simplest language we can, since in almost all the classical literature, it's always full of implication, metaphor, jargon and descriptions that are deliberately vague.

Taoists believe that yin and yang are united when the fetus is still in the womb. The spirit, which is energy, enters the new life (made of mother and father's vital essence) through the opening on top of the head. In the prenatal stage, yin and yang are perfectly balanced. At birth, upon the first breaths, life is separated from the original nature. Yin and yang are separated. Yin energy sinks down to the kidney, yang energy (pertaining to the mind) goes up to the heart, and spirit is housed inside the cavity behind the midpoint of the eyebrows. Once yin and yang are separated, they will gradually be out of balance due to the leakage of vital essence and spirit energy.

A perfectly united yin and yang is immortal. Once yin and yang become separated and imbalanced, mortal life begins.

The purpose of the Taoist alchemy is to return us to the state of the womb, uniting yin and yang. When the original yin (life force or sexual energy) is stirred, it is vital to circulate this energy upwards to let it unite with the yang energy, rather than letting it go downward out of the body, which is the natural course of expending life force.

Through alchemy, it is believed energy can become so pure that it results in an internal elixir.

Taoist internal or inner alchemy is a way of using your own body, mind and spirit in a quest for immortality.

This is different from Taoist's external alchemy, which is to search for immortality through various drugs, herbs and chemicals.

In more plain language, the basic premise of the esoteric Taoist internal alchemy is that we were born with a limited prenatal and postnatal vital life force, or chi. Through life activities, chi is gradually consumed and we ultimately die, as we discussed in Sections 7.5.1 and 7.5.3. Our chi or life force leaks through the process of orgasm with ejaculation in men and menstruation in women and through spiritual energy leaks as in Chapter 6. These are all activities that disperse chi or life force.

It is possible to turn life force inwards so that instead of losing chi, we use it to nourish and sustain our lives. It is also possible to actually absorb cosmic energies to enhance our life force. Once our cultivated life force is high and concentrated enough, we achieve what Taoists call the internal elixir, believed to be the ultimate immortality. More on immortality will be discussed in Chapter 10.

Taoism believes not only in spiritual development, but also in the longevity of the physical body. Therefore, alchemy of both body and spirit are required, This is because the longer you can sustain a vibrant physical body, the more time you have to perform alchemy for the ultimate goal of immortality. Thus, Taoism, if considered from a religious point of view, is the only religion that places so much emphasis on physical health and vitality.

The Taoist internal alchemy involves a large number of diversions in the ways it is practiced. It also encompasses many aspects and branches. But they all converge at essentially the same end point. It is many roads leading to the same destination.

The actual attainment of high-level practice of Taoist Alchemy is very individual. You must find your own way through your body, mind and spirit, since each of us is so different. You can only feel and sense it. You won't be able to describe it fully.

We have already touched some basics of Taoist internal alchemy. For example, the microcosmic and chi-gong state meditation discussed in Sections 5.3 and 6.4.1 can all be considered part of the alchemy. In PingLongevity™ Hormone, we will cover the parts that help conserve sexual energy.

The framework of Taoist internal alchemy for sexual energy can be summarized into the following principles.

7.5.4.1 Stimulation of Life Force

Stimulation of sexual energies increases our major hormone production and activates hormone receptors.

The best way to do this is through any sexual or non-sexual activities that excite your sexual energy.

This may also be done subconsciously, for example, during morning involuntary erections in men and in the days prior to menstruation in women, when there are signs of energy excitement. Usually women feel restless, dizzy, tired, or drowsy and have low back and leg soreness, swollen breasts, loss of appetite or a heavy feeling in the lower abdominal area.

Taoists consider this as the "raw materials" from which we can develop higher energies through alchemy.

Once you know how to collect sexual energies, you should stimulate sexual energy as much and as often as you can.

7.5.4.2 Collecting Life Force

Recall that chi or life force is a collection of life-sustaining prenatal and postnatal substances (hormones and blood) and higher energies (Section 7.5.1).

Once chi is awakened (Section 7.5.4.1), we must channel this very precious vital essence to nourish every cell of our bodies inwardly instead leaking it through orgasm with ejaculation (men) or menstruation (women).

You may ask, isn't it a natural process for males to leak semen in sexual activities and females to leak blood in menstruation? Isn't it nature's design to program life's clock to gradually consume life energy toward death? What can we do about it? Does preserving sexual energy mean reducing sexual pleasure?

We cannot control nature's course. After all, sex in humans is not just a reproductive activity; it is also for enjoyment. How can we avoid it? Besides, there is no way to change a woman's menstrual period.

In fact, we are able to change this natural process and simultaneously increase enjoyment. The purpose in doing so is to refine and transmute our sexual energy (the raw materials) to a better hormone level and to increase spirit energy, leading to extended youth, vital health and longevity. This reverses nature's course. There is an old Taoist saying, "For death, follow the flow of life; for life, reverse the flow of life."

How is this done? It can be done through chi-gong. In Section 5.3, we have quoted many studies that prove your mind can control your physical body.

We often ask people to do a simple experiment. Sit still, calm your mind and close your eyes. Place your hands palms up on your knees. Focus your attention on the middle of your palms. What do you feel? Pretty soon, you'll feel warmth and tingling. What is that? Your mind has "worked" chi and blood toward wherever it concentrates. So is this imaginary? Absolutely not! It is real.

Now think of the hormone testosterone in men. In Section 7.5.2, we quoted studies about increased sex hormone production with sexual activities. What if we can mentally direct the hormones to every part of our bodies, nourishing and revitalizing our entire systems? Think about the huge health benefit!

Physically, through chi-gong, we circulate hormones and blood into every corner of the body, which normally could have been stagnant, and thereby we activate the hormone receptors to maximize the health impact. On the spiritual plane, we use the "raw material" to develop higher energy (Chapter 10).

For men, it is important to appreciate the difference between orgasm and ejaculation.

What is the difference between having five ejaculations (and thus five orgasms) a week as compared with five orgasms a day without ever ejaculating? You're able to maximize the sex benefit and at the same time conserve life force.

Dr. John C. Lilly, at the National Institute of Neurological Diseases and Blindness, conducted a neurological study of monkeys in the 1950s that remains important to this day. He discovered points in the brain that control the sexual response of male monkeys.

Lilly also found that the neural points are different for different sexual functions. One neural point regulates arousal (erection). A second point regulates the orgasm itself (sensation of sexual peak and bliss of maximal satisfaction). The third point regulates muscular contraction (ejaculation).

The first and the second neural points control the pleasure, or entertainment aspects of sexual activities. The third one controls the reproductive aspect of sexual activity, i.e., ejaculation of sperm to give new life. In the usual course of life, we combine all three activities as though they must go together. Thus we limit ourselves in the enjoyment (because we cannot continuously ejaculate) and we pay the price of expending chi to build the potent semen.

Other research also indicates that stimulation of the septum, a portion of the brain known to be a part of the limbic system, results in the sensation of an orgasm, but this stimulation produces neither an erection nor ejaculation. These findings support the theory that ejaculation and orgasm, though often linked, are indeed separate events.

A 1992 National Health and Social Life Survey discovered that only 29% of women have orgasms every time they have sexual intercourse, compared to 75% of men who always have orgasms (and ejaculations). On the other hand, about 40% of both men and women said they are extremely emotionally satisfied with their experiences of sexual intercourse. Thus ejaculation and pleasure from sex are not all the same. They are controlled by different parts of the brain.

Although Lilly did not try to apply this research to human beings, his discovery indicates that it is possible, through conscious and learned control, for us to completely separate the entrainment center of the process of erection (circulatory system) and orgasm (neural system) from the mechanics of ejaculation (muscular system). If we can separate the two purposes of sexual activity, we can indeed maximize pleasure and minimize aging.

Before we proceed in circulating and transmuting the sexual energy, one caution must be kept in mind. In most people, energy meridians, or even physical channels such as the network of veins, have many blockages and extensive stagnation. In this case, chi cannot circulate adequately. That is why many times we need acupuncture to help open the blockages.

If we send a strong burst of chi through the body, for example the sexual energy, without leaking it, we may create a side effect if the sexual energy is stagnated in various parts of the body instead of smoothly circulating. This is what chi-gong masters talk about being "possessed by the evil" in many chi-gong exercises, meaning this stagnated energy may cause strange behaviors and even health problems.

Thus you must satisfy the prerequisite prior to freely circulating the energy:

• Completely opened microcosmic orbit (Section 5.4)

• Be able to achieve the chi-gong state (Section 6.4.1)

Circulating Sexual Energy: When chi is aroused, as discussed in Section 7.5.4.1, sexual energy is like a huge concentrated ball of condensed energy, like an unreleased atomic bomb. In fact, physically, as we discussed in Section 7.5.3, there is an increase of sex hormone levels and heightened brain dopamine level.

During such a situation, you should enter a chi-gong state as discussed in Section 6.4.1, however, instead of expanding yourself to the size of the universe, you keep within your boundary of your body. Disperse the ball of sexual energy into your entire body.

Rapid breathing and accelerated heartbeat are typical signs of sexual excitement. If you could achieve the chi-going state during sexual excitement, you should be able to keep your breathing very calm, light and slow, while your continue the sexual or sensual activities. For men, you should be able to achieve many orgasms without ejaculation.

7.5.4.3 Storing the Energy

In Chinese, *Tan* means "elixir" and *Tien* means "field." Elixir in Taoist alchemy means a highly refined concentrated form of immortal energy. Taoists believe that the practice of Taoist alchemy can ultimately result in the formation of an internal elixir that is so high it can sustain life indefinitely. This energy can create longevity and immortality.

Men has three Tan Tiens: the lower Tan Tien inside the naval where the prenatal vital essence is housed; the middle Tan Tien midway between the naval and the midpoint of the nipples, where the prenatal chi is stored; and the upper Tan Tien between the eyebrows and approximately one-third into the head, where the original spirit is housed.

Women also have three Tan Tiens: upper Tan Tien of Tanzhong midpoint between the nipples; middle Tan Tien, inside the navel; and lower Tan Tien, between the pubic bone and the navel corresponding to the ovaries.

The full extent of Taoist alchemy runs very deep and far. It is impossible to cover it all here. You should keep in mind, however, that yin energy accumulated from the stirring of the sexual essence can be vaporized through meditation and drawn upward into middle and upper Tan Tiens, where the yin energy, or sexual essence, copulates with the yang energy of the original chi and spirit and they are upgraded into higher energy. When this resulting energy due to the combination of yin and yang becomes large and dense, it becomes the elixir of immortality. The chi-gong state (Section 7.5.4.2) serves the purpose of the energy copulation. Now we are collecting the energy.

For men, towards the end of the practice, gradually focus your mind on Tan Tien (inside the naval). Condense all of this energy into the Tan Tien. Remain with your focus on the Tan Tien until you feel settled completely.

For women who do not need to conceive children, lightly focus (notice) on the Tanzhong cavity (midpoint between the nipples). Use both hands to smoothly massage the breasts in upward and outward circles. Do this for as long as you have time and feel comfortable. Then finally move your attention to the naval Tan Tien. Condense all the energy into the Tan Tien and remain with your focus there until you feel settled completely.

Women will notice that as you practice this meditation, your menstrual bleeding will decrease. In ancient Taoist alchemy, the goal is to return men and women to a pre-pubescent state. You will find your breasts become like a teenager's and your bleeding is slight. If you achieve this level of practice in middle age, you may delay menopause and minimize the symptoms.

For women who are still considering childbirth, simply focus on the Tan Tien to conclude each energy collection.

7.5.5   Improve Sexual Vitality

An added benefit of Taoist alchemy for transmuting sexual energy is that you can remain sexually active and virile for life.

Are you surprised at the popularity of Viagra? According to *Yahoo Health,* occasional impotence occurs "in about half of adult men in the U.S.; chronic impotence affects about one in eight American men."

Yahoo Health listed the following causes of impotence:

- Medication use (especially antihypertensives)

- Smoking

- Hormonal deficiency caused by disease (diabetes) or injury

- Liver disease, usually caused by alcoholism

- Circulation problems (arteriosclerosis, anemia, or vascular surgery)

- Neurological problems (injury, trauma, disease)

- Urological procedures (prostatectomy, orchiectomy, radiation therapy)

- Penile implants (or prostheses) that function improperly

- Depression, anxiety, fatigue, boredom, stress, fear of failure

- Mood-altering drugs, alcohol, medications

- Fear of infection

- Fear of recurring heart problems

- Deep-seated psychological problems

Keeping a youthful sex hormone level can cure many of the causes listed above. Taoist alchemy can help preserve this vitality.

7.5.6   Preventing Involuntary Leaks

For men, the morning involuntary erection is the time of your most potent sexual energy, unrelated to the workings of the mind. It is nature's design for a natural energy peak cycle, a measure of your health and vitality. If you do not have early morning erections, this is a sure sign of a weakened body system.

All men have a daily cycle of testosterone levels that peak somewhere between 4 and 6 A.M., coinciding with the time when many men have early morning erections. These involuntary erections are a normal part of the sleep cycle for most men and, according to research, most men have perhaps three or four of these cycles each night. There are various theories as to why nature planned it this way: One suggests that this is a way the male penis "renews" itself with an ample supply of oxygen.

In the celebrated I Ching, the ancient sages divided the energy cycle of each day according to the waxing and waning of yin and yang energies. Between 9 and 11 P.M. is the extreme of yin energy. Yang energy starts to emerge between 11 P.M. and 1 A.M., and reaches its maximum between 7 and 9 A.M. Therefore Taoists believe the early morning erection corresponds to the peak yang energy in the body. If sexual energy is the most potent energy, its peak is even more potent. Men must take advantage of this peak energy as the raw materials to refine into higher energy.

Wet dreams are quite unconscious events. Most of the time when we awaken, ejaculation has already occurred. Therefore, if you have a history of frequent wet dreams, you should perform chi-gong in any form such as the ones covered in Sections 5.4 or 6.4.1 before sleep to calm the mind and energy and thus prevent the sexual energy leakage.

7.6   FOOD HORMONE THERAPY

While there are many specific foods that are good for hormone balance, it is most important to follow the PingLongevity™ Diet, for the significant benefit of regulating the glucose control axis (Section 7.2.4), and PingLongevity™ Caloric Restriction protocols, for postponing the entire aging process to retain youthful hormones (Section 3.3.6).

7.6.1   Foods for Men

For men, usually the age-related imbalance is estrogen dominance (Section 7.2.5), which results in many degenerative diseases. The key is to increase the production of testosterone, inhibit the conversion of testosterone to DHT and to estrogen and enhance liver's capability to eliminate extra estrogen.

The following foods and substances are to be considered:

- Examples of testosterone-enhancing foods are: venison, shrimp, prawns, lobster, deer kidneys, pigeon, pigeon eggs, beef kidney, mussels, kelp, chestnuts, lamb, cinnamon, leeks, celery, green onions, onions, garlic, raw oysters, bananas, almonds and avocadoes.

- Examples of foods that help reduce testosterone to estrogen conversion are: broccoli, cabbage, cauliflower, Brussels sprouts, kale and bok choy.

- Some liver detoxification foods are: mung beans, carrots, beets, garlic, tomatoes, brazil nuts, asparagus, watermelon, papaya, avocado, spinach, eggs, broccoli, cayenne pepper, lemon and walnuts.

- Men should avoid grapefruit because it tends to inhibit the excretion of estrogen from the liver.

- Alcohol should also be avoided. Research has demonstrated that both acute and chronic alcohol exposure are associated with low levels of hypothalamic LHRH and pituitary LH in the adult and pubertal male rat. Further studies have suggested that alcohol inhibits testosterone secretion by the testes as well.

- Drugs, such as Lipitor and other statin drugs, anti-histamines, anti-psychotics, narcotics, anti-fungals, anti-convulsants, blood pressure medications and recreational drugs, all lower androgen levels, so they should be avoided as much as possible.

7.6.2   Foods for Women

For women, estrogen dominance is most often the problem, despite the sharp drop of estrogen at menopause (Section 7.2.5).

The following foods are good for hormone balancing in women:

- Foods containing phytoestrogens such as isoflavones are found in soybeans, licorice, kudzu, alfalfa, black cohosh and red clover. They act both on the estrogen receptors as well as on the enzymes that metabolize them. Certain isoflavones are also natural cancer-protective compounds.

- Foods with lignans, found in many fruits and seeds, produce a compound that triggers the excretion of estrogen in the urine, decreasing the amount of estrogen in the body and inhibiting its ability to influence hormone-dependent diseases. Studies show that breast cancer rates are lower in women who excrete higher amounts of lignans in their urine.

- Foods with coumestans, such as alfalfa and red clover help to balance estrogen levels by triggering estrogenic activity when estrogen levels are low and by competing for estrogen receptor binding sites when estrogen levels are high. High and low estrogen levels can impact mood swings and hot flashes.

- Foods that naturally increase progesterone are sweet potatoes, wild yam, egg yolks and dairy products, shellfish, curry, thyme and oregano.

- Like men, women should also use liver cleansing foods such as mung beans, carrots, beets, garlic, tomatoes, Brazil nuts, asparagus, watermelon, papaya, avocado, spinach, eggs, broccoli, squash, cayenne pepper, lemon and walnuts.

7.6.3   The Myth of Tofu

Media reports have confused many of us about the health value of tofu. They say erroneously that eating tofu can cause female sex characteristics in men due to its phytoestrogen content. This is particularly harmful when popular doctors also promote this myth. There are even articles that claim "soy makes kids gay."

Scientific studies have conflicting results. Some support the benefit of soy, while others showed negative results.

Is phytoestrogen good or bad? Soy products and particularly tofu have been consumed in Japan, China and other Asian countries for thousands of years. Why is it suddenly condemned by modern medicine and Western countries?

What the studies and media do not seem to understand is that phytoestrogen, the plant estrogen that resides in soy products, can dilute or enhance your body's estrogen.

On one hand, phytoestrogen is estrogen-like in the sense that it occupies estrogen receptors and has a weak estrogenic effect. The good thing about phytoestrogen is that it occupies estrogen receptors where it would be otherwise seized by stronger estrogens produced by your own body. Therefore, it reduces the dominant estrogen effect in aging.

However, on the other hand, if you flood your body with too much phytoestrogen, you may have more receptors filled that otherwise would be empty. In this case, it gives rise to more estrogenic effect! So you can see, it is all about balance!

In hormone therapies, sometimes you want to dilute, while other times you want to enhance your own body's estrogenic effects. So when using concentrated forms of phytoestrogen supplements, you need to really know what you are doing, as discussed in Section 7.3.

In whole foods like soybeans and tofu, it's very difficult to overdose. Therefore the myth about tofu and whole food soy is not correct.

7.7   NATURAL HORMONE BALANCING

By natural hormone balancing, we mean therapies using natural supplements and herbs, rather than the use of real hormones either synthetic or bio-identical. This is a less potent way of hormone balancing and replacement than real hormone therapies. However, as we discussed in Section 2.8.1, even natural supplements have risks due to the potency and high concentrations made possible by modern technologies. Therefore, you must know what to do to avoid the risk of side effects from tinkering with hormones (Section 7.3).

7.7.1   Natural Hormone Balancing for Men

As mentioned in Section 7.6.1, we attempt to increase the production of testosterone, inhibit the conversion of testosterone to DHT and estrogen and to enhance the liver's capability to eliminate excess estrogen:

- Examples of TCM formulas or dietary supplements that use high concentrations of one or a combination of the following ingredients help increase testosterone: tiger penis, snake penis, wolfberry fruit, curculigo, dodder, cynomorium, epimedium, velvet, psoralen, morinda, ginseng, kowloon, cordyceps sinensis, actinolite and royal jelly.

- TCM formulas, Wu Zi Zong Yang and Jin Gui Shen Qi help increase testosterone levels.

- Whey protein can be used to increase growth hormone, which in turn enhances the production of testosterone.

- Zinc supplementation inhibits levels of the testosterone to estrogen conversion enzyme aromatase.

- Dietary supplements from high concentration extracts of resveratrol, milk thistle, cruciferous vegetables (e.g., broccoli, cauliflower, cabbage, and Brussels sprouts) and TCM formulas such as Long Dan Xie Gan and Jia Wei Xiao Yao improve the liver's ability to excrete excess estrogen.

- Dietary supplements from high concentration extracts of saw palmetto and stinging nettle, as well as the prescription drug Propecia can be used to inhibit 5-alpha reductase, the enzyme to convert testosterone to DHT (Section 7.2.5).

- Iodine supplementation is very important for sex hormone balance. Most people are deficient in iodine. The reason may be that our water has too much chlorine and our bakeries, too much bromide, both competing with iodine by flushing iodine from the body. When we are deficient in iodine, the metabolism slows and people become overweight. Fat tissue produces estrogen and estrogen dominance occurs.

> "Now I see more and more men having erectile dysfunction problems, starting even in their late 30s and early 40s. We usually start with detoxifying the liver, which will balance the hormones and excrete excess estrogens, increase the kidney energy and promote blood circulation. We have seen good responses."
>
> —Dr. Ping

7.7.2   Natural Hormone Balancing for Women

For females, estrogen dominance is also the most common problem, despite the sharp drop of estrogen at menopause (Section 7.2.5). Our purpose is not only to increase estrogen, but to increase progesterone even more in order to balance the ratio. For many menopausal women, additional testosterone may be also needed:

- Dietary supplements containing phytoestrogen extracts from soy, red clover and flaxseed, as well as herbs such as black cohosh, dong quai and wolfberry can help increase estrogen production and balance female hormones.

- Supplements of wild yam help increasing progesterone.

- The TCM formula Jia Wei Xiao Yao works to reduce estrogen dominance.

- The Chinese herb epimedium can help increase testosterone.

- Like men, women need to cleanse their livers. Dietary supplements from high concentration extracts of resveratrol, milk thistle, cruciferous vegetables (e.g. broccoli, cauliflower, cabbage and Brussel sprouts) and TCM formulas such as Long Dan Xie Gan improve the liver's ability to excrete excess estrogen.

- Like men, women should use iodine supplementation.

> "I've seen so many women stop their periods in their late 30s and early 40s. Debbie, 34 years old, had no periods for two years. Doctors prescribed birth control pills, which brought her period back for two months, then it died out even though she continued on the pill. She and her husband want to have children, so she came to my office seeking natural ways to address her problem. We reduced her stress patterns, rebalanced her adrenals, cleansed her liver, balanced her estrogen/progesterone through natural herbs and supplements, as well as acupuncture. After two months, she returned to regular periods and soon after she naturally conceived. Now her baby is three years old."
>
> —Dr. Ping

> "50-year-old Jasmine's period stopped when she was 38. She had all the symptoms of menopause: night sweats, hot flashes, dry skin and loss of sex drive. By clearing her liver toxins, increasing her kidney energy and revitalizing her ovaries, her period returned and now in her 50s, she has regular periods. Her sex life was revitalized, too. People comment how beautiful she looks. She thinks she looks younger than when she was 38."
>
> —Dr. Ping

7.8   SUMMARY

We can summarize the main points of this chapter as the follows:

- Hormones have a fundamental role in aging. As you age, most of your hormones decline and become imbalanced. This is the root cause of many degenerative diseases such as heart disease, obesity, cancer, depression, osteoporosis and diabetes. Therefore, keeping a youthful hormone level is fundamentally important.

- Although you must address your hormone problems in order to stay youthful and vibrant, it can be risky to tinker with hormones through hormone balance and replacement therapies if you don't know the correct ways. You must find a doctor who truly understands the intricacies of hormones.

- You must baseline your hormone levels as close to the ages of 18 to 22 years of age as you can, or when you are still young and vibrant, so you can determine your own individualized optimal hormone level. The exception to the 18- to 22-year optimal hormone target rule is for sex hormones of perimenopausal and menopausal women, as well as DHT for men.

- To address hormonal imbalances, lifestyle approaches such as diet, caloric restriction and food therapy should be your first choices. Then use natural herb and dietary supplement hormone balance and replacement therapy. As a last resort, you may choose to use bio-identical hormone replacement therapies to be discussed in Chapter 9.

CHAPTER 8

Look and Act Young

Although in this chapter, we'll talk about how to look young, it is very important to remember that if you want to look young from the outside, you must be young from the inside in the first place by practicing PingLongevity™ discussed in the previous chapters.

We can easily see the relationship between the outside and the inside. Skin elasticity (Section 1.2.1) is one of the true biomarkers of aging. It demonstrates not only how the skin ages, but how your entire being ages. Just pinch the skin on the back of your hand between your thumb and forefinger for five seconds and see how long it takes to return to normal. This will take less than 1 second for people in their 20s as compared with 10 to 15 seconds for a 60-year-old. Therefore, before you pay so much money for expensive cosmetics and plastic surgery, you must live a lifestyle that will promote whole body health. This will have a much more dramatic effect on how you look on the surface! This is not something a cream or a surgery can do.

Assuming that you are on a clean healthy diet, practice caloric restriction to delay aging, do functional fitness, connect your body with your mind and maintain a youthful hormone level, now we can discuss some of the skin-deep methods of keeping a young look.

PingLongevity ™ Look believes keeping a younger look is very important psychologically to maintain high self-confidence as you age. High confidence gives you a positive mental reinforcement, which in turn stimulates the vitality of the physical body. This is a positive cycle of life enhancement and is absolutely necessary for your overall well-being.

8.1   VIBRANT SKIN FOR LIFE

Maintaining healthy skin is an important part of longevity, not just for a youthful look but because the skin is a very important organ of the body, responsible for many respiratory functions. Skin protects us from environmental changes, cold, heat, wind, injury and disease. Occasionally you meet someone who looks to be 40 but is actually 60 and you wonder, "Why?"

8.1.1   Photo-Aging: the Biggest Skin Destroyer

"Have you wondered why the skin on your face, neck, hands, forearms—the places most exposed to the sun—look a lot older than, for example, the skin on your buttocks?

Many times, when you stand in line waiting for cashiers, you may have noticed that people in front of you have necks, shoulders and faces full of sun spots, wrinkles, deep lines and other signs of skin aging, even though they are still relatively young. Is the short-term pleasure of being in the sun worth this permanent damage?"

—DR. PING

Sun exposure is the most common cause of skin damage, but this is a complex subject. On one hand, most of us know that we need sunlight to get vitamin D for bone health and many other health benefits. Sun exposure also gives us

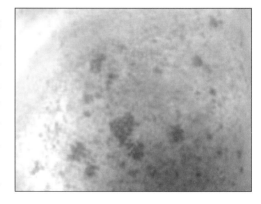

a tanned healthy look, a symbol of the wealthy and leisurely lifestyle. Corporate executives like to have suntans, simply to demonstrate that they have a great life outside of work despite their busy schedules.

On the other hand, the sun's ultraviolet rays are the most damaging to the skin. Let's look at scientific studies. Ultraviolet rays consist of a wide spectrum of energy. The shorter the wavelength, the more energy it carries. Life on earth can tolerate only a small portion of the wide spectrum of ultraviolet waves. Humans can naturally see and feel a small portion of the light spectrum from the sun. We see colors at the low end of the spectrum; we sense the warmth of the infrared light energy. But the rest of the sun's powerful waves, like X-rays or ultraviolet waves, surround us unnoticed.

Ultraviolet (UV) light waves are the most damaging to human skin. UV light also has several different wavelengths. The longest wavelengths penetrate deepest into the skin and cause the most potential damage. When sunlight hits the skin, it is absorbed by a type of pigment called melanin. Melanin is what makes our skin dark, both naturally and after sun exposure. The amount of melanin determines our natural skin color, so Caucasians have very little melanin and Africans have a great deal of melanin. This pigment protects the genetic machinery of our cells by absorbing sunlight and turning the skin darker, making it tan. Severe sun exposure will cause a lack of sufficient protection the melanin pigment. The lighter our natural skin color, the harder it is to protect ourselves from the sun.

Many of us are exposed not only to direct sunlight, but also to various forms of UV light. For example, so-called "black lights" or UV lamps are used to kill bacteria in the food processing industry. We also treat acne under UV lights. Now we employ tanning beds, which use UV light to produce an artificial tan.

There are several sub-spectrums within UV light—UVA, UVB, UVC. UVA has the longest wavelength of the three. UVC is normally filtered out entirely by the earth's atmosphere, so the main impact on us comes from UVA and UVB.

Many people believe that UVA is safe. For example, tanning bed operators use UVA light and claim it does not damage the skin. Most sunscreens are rated by sun protection factor (SPF) numbers that refer only to the effect of UVB radiation because UVA is assumed to be safe.

The fact is that both UVA and UVB are damaging. Thus, using artificial UVA tanning lights or sunscreens may not protect us from skin damage.

UVB radiation has long been considered the root cause of sunburn. Exposure to UVB causes a burning sensation quickly and leaves an initial reddish cast to the skin. Delayed tanning occurs several days after the initial exposure as a result of increased activity or increased production of melanin stimulated by the UVB exposure.

UVA, on the other hand, does not burn the skin directly, but it does produce an immediate tan, which is why tanning beds are so popular. The majority of solar ultraviolet radiation that reaches the earth's surface is UVA. This is why conventional wisdom claims that UVA is safe. Unfortunately, it is becoming increasingly clear that no UV exposure is safe. UVA can penetrate deep into the skin, causing damage to DNA and leading to wrinkling, spotting and skin cancers that we wrongly attribute to normal aging. UVA also injures blood vessels, causing the broken capillaries often seen on the nose and cheeks of sun-damaged individuals. UVA can also burn the eyes, resulting in cataracts over time.

Eventually a suntan recedes, giving the impression that any damage done is gone forever. But the damage is a lot deeper. As we age, our systems simply cannot repair or replace all the damaged cells deep below the surface of the skin. The accumulation of this damage accelerates aging. Thus, both UVA and UVB exposure create significant skin damage. There is no safe exposure, even to UVA rays only.

Not only is skin damaged from UV light due to insufficient melanin protection, but sunlight intensifies the oxidation process. As we discussed earlier, skin cells live best in a moist, low oxygen concentration environment. Sunlight bakes out the natural and applied oil of the skin and dries the natural moisture layer. Think of frying an egg in an oiled pan. The heat will dry up the oil and fry the egg. Similarly, we often see older people on the beach with their skin hanging like dried paper folds, baking in the sun's "frying pan." They have parched their skin and oxidized it to the maximum. Long-term UV exposure intensifies skin oxidation.

So what is wrong with beaten-up skin if we can exchange it for the joy of the suntan and the fun? It makes a world of difference from a longevity point of view. We want you not only to be much younger than your peer group from biological, physiological and spiritual points of view, but also to look 20 years younger than they do. Dry, weathered and wrinkled skin on the face, neck, lower arms and hands will make you look extremely old, especially after your 40s.

We have a little more leeway to expose more of ourselves to the sun as children, at least until the age of 15. This is because we have a high ability to repair the damaged skin cells and regenerate new ones when we are very young. When we get older, the ability to repair the damage is diminished. So we can fix some damage and other damage becomes permanent.

You may ask that if we stay totally out of the sun, how we can still have a life? You definitely can. Here's what you need to do: Try to avoid direct sunlight completely—all the time—since most sunscreen simply will not protect you. When you must be in the sun, wear a hat, long sleeves and long pants, and cover your hands, if possible. Even if you are completely covered, if you are near water, or where lots of reflection occurs, you need to wear zinc oxide-based sunscreen, which offers the most protection.

Avoiding direct sunlight does not have to deter you from outdoor activities. You can go rafting, hiking, boating, swimming, traveling, etc. Some sports and activities can be done indoors (such as swimming) or in the early morning or after sunset and during the evening hours (such as surfing).

If you really do want to have a suntan, there are many tanning creams and sprays that give you a tan without having to expose yourself to sunlight or tanning beds.

How we can be sure to have enough vitamin D, which is so essential to our bones and to our hormonal systems? To get enough vitamin D from the sun, we need to be exposed to direct sunlight,

UVB rays, about 30 minutes twice a week. Notice that we are talking about being outside on a clear day, with little pollution, with no sunscreen and with an exposed face, shoulders, back, legs and arms. This is enough to create sun damage to the skin. Therefore, the best way is to take enough vitamin D from foods such as fish and fish oil and to use dietary supplements. The PingLongevity™ Test (Section 1.4) includes regular vitamin D testing.

8.1.2   Skin Protection Methods

Besides using zinc oxide-based sunscreens when you're outside (even without direct sunlight), what is the best cream for skin protection? Every day, you can find dozens of new products on the market. You buy them and before long, those creams and potions and lotions have overwhelmed your bathroom counters.

To understand which cream is best for skin protection, you must understand that skin thrives under low oxygen conditions and likes oil-based topical protection.

A series of important experiments has shown how oxygen influences cellular growth and life span. It was found that oxygen is actually detrimental to cell growth. Fresh sea level room air, or most of the environment we live in, contains about 20% oxygen, which is not the most optimal environment for cell growth. Most types of skin cells, whether for simple growth or to heal wounds, grow best at oxygen levels similar to those carried inside the body, about 1–2% oxygen. At such low oxygen concentration, cells not only grow faster, but, contradictory to popular belief, they live longer.

If we apply a little common sense, it is not hard to understand the results of such experiments. We all know how oxygen oxidizes metal. That is how brown-colored copper turns green. This is how metal structures turn rusty. When we cut vegetables and fruits, they become oxidized at the site of the cut, forming a brown-colored layer. In fact, the free radical theory says that aging is due to oxidants combining with DNA and other body structures such as proteins to form derivatives. Over time, these free radicals degenerate the body systems.

Another simple observation is to compare people living in warm and humid climates with people in dry places. All other factors being equal (especially the amount of sun exposure), people living in warm, humid places tend to have better skin. This is because their skin is constantly covered with the sweat and oil that the body secretes as well as moisture in the air, which seal off the impact of oxygen attack. Their skin cells live longer and regenerate faster when they are damaged. On the other hand, people living in dry places tend to have weathered skin that makes them look older than their chronological age. *Thus, a simple basic principle for maintaining a youthful look: Skin lives longer and heals quicker in a very low oxygen environment of less than 1 to 2% oxygen.*

The free radical theory of aging is another major discovery in skin aging. It is well known that the cells generate free radical byproducts in the process of consuming energy. These are unstable oxygen molecules. Free radicals can attach themselves to other atoms and molecules, such as proteins, causing general aging. A less-known discovery is that most of the damage by free radicals is in the outer layer of the cell, called the cell plasma membrane, rather than the interior of the cell, such as cellular DNA. The free radicals are drawn to areas that have the greatest density of molecules in the outer layers. Once the cell's outer layer is damaged, it becomes inefficient at letting nutrients in and letting waste out (for example, salt). As a result, the cell becomes dehydrated and looks old. The outer layer of the cell is mostly fat. Most anti-aging facial creams are water-soluble rather than fat-soluble, because the conventional wisdom is that the free-radical damage occurs in the interior of the cell that is water-soluble. *Thus, it's important to use an oil soluble anti-oxidant cream, which can penetrate into the outer layer of the skin cell.*

Now if you seal your skin with a high quality oil-based cream, you can count on younger looking skin look over time!

8.1.3 Wrinkles and Lines

Wrinkles and lines are mostly formed where frequent folding of skin is required, such as the side of the eyes (crow's feet), forehead wrinkles (frown or squint lines), neck lines, hand lines, stomach lines, etc.

You'll have to take extra care of these places with more frequent application of oil-based moisturizers as discussed in Section 8.1.2.

You should also avoid bad posture. For example, many people have deep lines on the backs of their necks. This is because they slump in their regular standing posture so that their heads have to rise upwards, causing a crease in the neck. Lines on the back of the hands are due to certain repetitive movements, for example, long-term typing on the computer with bent wrists. Both can be corrected by improved posture.

Botox™ is a good technique to use to lessen crow's feet and forehead wrinkles. It not only makes the wrinkles disappear, but also prevents the wrinkles from becoming deeper. This is because wrinkles and lines are formed by frequent bending or folding of the skin. Just get a piece of cloth. If you fold it in one place many times, over time, you'll see that a crease will form.

Many people are against Botox™. First, they think the remedy is temporary because they are unaware of the preventive effect of avoiding skin folds. Second, they think about the poisoning effects of the components of the drug. Yes, indeed, botulinum toxin type A is a protein produced by the bacterium *clostridium botulinum,* and is known to be extremely neurotoxic. However, it's been widely used, and side effects occur only to a very small percent of people and those are usually minor. Considering the preventive nature, we are not against using Botox™.

If you choose to use Botox™, you need to choose a good professional to administer it because, like any other aesthetic procedure, it is not only a medical procedure, but also an art form. Not all doctors are artists. Some can make you look unnatural.

Another much-overlooked cause of skin wrinkles is the fast and feast cycle when people lose and gain weight in a short period of time through the fad weight loss programs. Many people periodically go on diets. These weight loss programs range from strict fasting on fruit juice only to powdered supplements. Most of the time, we lose a few pounds and quickly gain them back when we return to a normal routine. Seldom are people willing to live on such programs forever and completely change the lifestyle that made them fat in the first place. As a result, they go through fast and feast cycles, becoming fat, then thin, then fat again. As we age, our skin gradually loses elasticity. It does not shrink automatically when we reduce in size. Therefore our skin hangs in many folds as the fat is lost. So an added benefit of keeping a constant adult life weight is to reduce the drama on the skin.

8.1.4 Skin Rejuvenation and Maintenance

Once a while, you need to regularly maintain your skin. Included in maintenance is the removal of small skin tags and growths that can be easily removed by electric needles.

You need to rejuvenate your skin periodically. There are many methods and just as many pros and cons, such as chemical peel, laser resurfacing, pulsed light resurfacing. You'll need to do this because your body loses the ability to completely renew the aged skin cells on the surface as you age. It also lost some ability to hold onto water, collagen and fat. By rejuvenation, you stimulate cell growth.

In general, we prefer the rejuvenation procedures that are less invasive and require essentially no down time. One simple procedure we prefer is to use a micro needle roller, a roller with hundreds of acupuncture like needles, to stimulate the skin, e.g., face, hands and neck. You may choose to apply anesthetic cream first to minimize pain. This will create injury sites to mobilize the body's repair mechanisms (stem cells) and to stimulate the body's growth capability. Since you have created many micro holes in your skin, you may use skin nutrition to intensify the repair. Stem cell growth factors and cytokines show good results in combination with micro needle rollers, more to be discussed in Chapter 9.

Another effective method is to use high frequency energy, cold laser light emitting micro-current, color, harmonic sound and gemstone devices. This class of treatment devices has the effect of cleaning up the lymphatic system and removing toxins from the body. It is also great for repairing rosacea, acne, sun damage and other skin disorders. It can stimulate the cellular growth of collagen.

8.1.5   Self Care Regimen for Younger Skin

Other self-care tips include the following simple steps:

- Drink two glass of alkaline ionized water on an empty stomach first thing in the morning to detoxify your lymphatic system and reduce your overnight acid production.

- Gently massage the face promoting blood circulation. One method is to lightly pat the face using your fingertips, especially around eye areas, cheek and around the mouth.

- Cleanse the skin well using natural nano silver soap, which kills 99% of bacteria.

- Apply a natural oil moisturizer, such as small molecule easy penetrating elastin and collagen, as well as human stem cell growth factor serums.

- Take multi-vitamins, minerals, fish oil and collagen.

8.2   POSTURE AND RIGIDITY

Unless you have severe osteoporosis, there is really no excuse for you to have poor posture. The most frequently seen postural problems are: flat back (standing with no curvature at the lower back), slouching (sit tilted without support on the lower back) and hunchback.

These postures are not only will cause problems in your lower back and neck, but also make you look old. You must consciously correct your posture on a day-to-day basis.

You may have noticed that some people, when they get older, tend to have a very rigid posture. It is as though their upper bodies are one piece without movement above the hips. This may be due to physical reasons, such as when all the discs between the bones deteriorate, making it difficult for the body to move spinal fluid. However, we believe that for many people, it's also a mindset. When they accept the notion that they are getting old, they begin to act old. They should look at how young people walk. Poor posture is only partially due to a lack of capability. So it's important that you make an effort to act young because then you'll look young.

8.3   HEALTHY TEETH

Good healthy teeth are symbol of good health. They are also a part of overall youthful look. Are you allowing yourself to have yellowed teeth, infected gums, bad breath and eventually lose all of your teeth and the need for dentures? With proper regular maintenance, teeth can be kept healthy for life.

Regular dental maintenance requires a few simple steps: brush teeth at least twice a day; floss or use a water jet to clean teeth daily before bedtime; have a professional cleaning quarterly or bi-annually, as well as annual checkups for cavities, gum disease and cancer.

This is very simple step, but it's surprising how many people neglect their teeth.

8.4   FAT REDISTRIBUTION

"For one thing, we should realize that one of the main causes of aging is the apparent loss of fat in one's face. Typically, we think of the aging face as one in which the skin and underlying muscles have stretched in response to wear and tear and the effect of gravity. While this is true to some extent and can often be repaired with more traditional procedures, such as a face-lift, we find that the loss of fat may be an even greater contributor to the appearance of aging. If we only look at the round cheeks of a baby and compare that with the more hollowed appearance of an adult it is clear that there are tremendous changes in the distribution of fat. The skin may be thought of as an envelope and the underlying fat and muscles as the contents. As the contents thin out, then there will be a relatively larger envelope. In the case of the face, this will appear in the form of sagging or wrinkles. If we could replace fat in some of these areas, then we might be able to restore a more youthful and attractive appearance."

—DR. MARK BERMAN, PRESIDENT OF THE AMERICAN ACADEMY OF COSMETIC SURGERY

According to the procreation theory of aging in Section 1.3.1, the purpose of our existence is to procreate. Once the job is done, the body goes into a steep decline and we age and die.

Nature has also made it such that we look bad, too, as we age. One sure sign of aging is the redistribution of fat. Although aging generally results in increased weight and body fat, certain areas actually have less fat. The face, neck, hands and feet, in particular, lose volume of fat, while the middle sections in men and hips and thighs in women gain fat.

Since we are talking about how we look, let's focus on the face. Artists can draw a young and an older person with only a few lines. You can see that volume of fat in the face is lost around the mouth, making the area around the mouth sink. Fat is also lost around the cheeks, upper eyelids, eyebrows, lips and on the forehead. Because of this, the extra skin has no place to go but to hang down, creating a large line down from the nose to each side of the mouth, bags under the eyes, drooping of the outer lids of the eyes, wrinkly forehead and turkey neck. Overall, because of fat volume loss, the face begins to look like the underlying skeletal structure and wherever there is cavity, it sags into it.

Published in the *Journal of the American Society of Plastic Surgeons* in 2008, Dr. Sean Darcy et al, showed the following MRI images of a 21-year-old (left) and a 63-year-old (right). As you can see in the illustration on the next page, the younger person has much more fat (the white area under the eye) than the older.

A few years ago, facelifts became the big craze in cosmetics. Facelifts make money for plastic surgeons, but they create huge

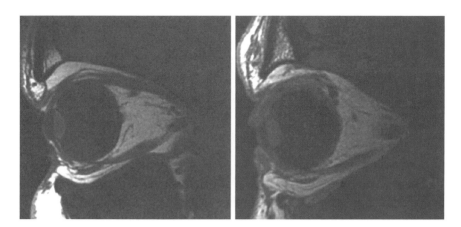

scars on the face and lift empty skin "envelope." As a result, it looks unnatural.

The recent trend is to use fillers instead, since many plastic surgeons have caught up with the idea of the lost volume of fat that contributes to a wrinkly, aged face. The problem is that most filler, such as Cosmoderm™, Zyderm™, Restylane™, use synthetic materials. They are artificial consumable materials and must be refilled in a few months. They are preferred methods because they cost doctors very little time and skill and guarantee return business. Unlike Botox™, they have no preventative impact. All they do is to temporarily fill in the space. Since they are foreign materials, they will ultimately be absorbed by the body. One worry we have is that they may act as a barrier for nutrients and repair mechanisms to reach the surface of the skin and they may create scar tissue underneath the skin.

Your own fat is the best filler of all, the fat that slipped down to you belly, hips or thighs. Although not verified, it's possible that fat in the belly is actually genetically programmed to remain there when you get older, and when transferred to the face, it may stay for life. Done properly, most fat grafted to the face, hands and neck may survive and remain for life.

Another advanced natural procedure is to spike stem cells of your own into the fat to be grafted. We'll discuss more of this procedure in Chapter 9.

8.5   HAIR REDISTRIBUTION

If fat redistribution isn't enough to make you look old, you also experience body hair redistribution as you age. Most of us, particularly men, lose hair density at the top and frontal portions of the head, eyebrows and eyelashes. You'll increase hair and hair length at the tip of eyebrows, nose and all body hair.

Almost all males lose hair at the crown of the head, so by the time you are middle aged, you usually have less than 50% of the density you had when you were in your teens, and many have receding hairlines. At 50% density, you really cannot see baldness. However, if you may notice how lush and thick a teenage boy's hair is. It is as though they have so much hair that there is not enough space on their heads to hold it all. That's the look of the lushness of 100% dense healthy hair.

Male pattern baldness is a more severe problem that affects many people who lose more than 70% of the hair on the top and temple area so that the baldness becomes very apparent.

The root cause of male pattern baldness is primarily due to a shift of hormone balance as we age. The ratio between testosterone, especially free testosterone, and dihydrotestosterone (DHT) will decrease. When testosterone combines with an enzyme called 5-alpha reductase, DHT is produced. DHT is believed to attack hair follicles and slowly shrinks them until they fall out and disappear completely. The ratio between testosterone and estrogen, which decreases as we age, has a significant impact on male pattern baldness.

There are ways to reduce male pattern baldness. For example, many herbs (Section 7.7) and drugs (Propecia) inhibit the conversion from testosterone to DHT and thus protect the hair follicles from being affected.

One important thing to notice is that the hair on the back of the head genetically keeps the high density it had during youth at about 100%. Somehow that portion of the hair carries the genetic message to stay, while the hair follicles on the top and front of the head are programmed to lose density. This is the basis of natural hair transplant. It's a proven procedure, without side effects, if done properly and artistically, to sample some hair follicles from the back of the head, and graft them to the top and frontal parts of the head. Properly implanted, the success rate is very high. This procedure is again highly dependent on the doctors' skill and artistry.

Besides hair grafting, there are a few other ways to promote hair growth, which have produced good results:

"In our clinic, we treat many people, men and women, with thinning hair. We found there are multiple underlying reasons for the problem. Fixing the root causes has given us good treatment results:

- Iodine deficiency: With supplementation, we can help maintain healthy thyroid function, which promotes hair growth.

- A lack of protein absorption: Use protein powder and essential amino acid supplementation. For example, Mary has a long-term problem absorbing proteins from foods. Tests showed a lack of essential amino acids. When protein was supplemented, she re-grew her formerly thick hair.

- A lack of key minerals such as silicon and iron.

- Estrogen/progesterone imbalance: When supplemented with progesterone, many female patients responded with improved scalp hair growth.

- DHT/testosterone imbalance: Using herbs and Propecia to reduce the conversion from testosterone to DHT helps prevent male patients' scalp hair from thinning.

- Additionally, stem cell growth factors have been found to stimulate hair growth."

—Dr. Ping

Thinning hair on your scalp and the frontal part of your head can sometimes be accompanied by increased hair growth in other parts of the body, such as the tips of the eyebrows, nose and ears.

8.6   YOUNG FASHION

In middle age, you may seldom notice how the young people dress, and how fashions change every year. Your own fashion sense may have become stale. You may be always picking up the same type of nice ties, collecting the same old style cut in suits and wearing the same types of clothing.

Although it may be required to remain conservative for most of your work life, to stay young, especially at heart, develop a fashion sense based on the fashions young people are wearing and adopt it, especially in a more casual setting. Don't be afraid to change your fashion personality. It will make you look and feel young.

8.7   BEING IN SYNC

One of the most telling signs of aging is being *out of the era*. The society is moving forward with new technology, new values, new trends and belief systems. If you cannot keep up with the times and be "hip" like the younger generations, you're behind the times. We have seen so many people who spend their lives stuck in the time frame of their 20s. So 30 years later, they are 30 years behind. And 50 years later, they are 50 years behind the times. They behave and act old-fashioned. The following is a list of signs that you are behind the times:

• Not knowing how to use e-mail;

• Cannot text message;

• Don't use the Internet;

• Cannot appreciate current pop music and culture;

• Cannot keep up conversations on current topics of interest to people of younger generations;

• Cannot keep up with the current state of politics, culture, events, law, belief, etc.

• Do not use a cell phone, especially more trendier and high tech models.

• Still only sing decades-old pop songs.

When you're out of the era, you are unconsciously behaving in an old-fashioned way. If you're too far out of this era, you're detached socially. You become ignored by the mainstream. You become redundant to the society. You become a non-contributor. This not only impacts your health, but your personal look and the way you present yourself.

8.8   SUMMARY

In this chapter, we discussed the "look and feel" side of living a youthful and healthy life. The PingLongevity ™ Look includes the following:

- The way you look and act is a major yardstick of youthfulness.

- Protect your skin from direct sun exposure, use good oil-based cream, minimize wrinkles and lines and perform skin rejuvenation periodically.

- Make a conscious effort to improve your posture, and especially not to slump and look like an old person.

- Maintaining healthy teeth is simple and easy, but you have to commit to daily dental hygiene and regular dental cleaning.

- Be aware of the methods of preventing and fixing fat and hair redistribution problems.

- Being in tune with the fashions of the younger generations so that you're not left behind.

- Be in sync with the changes in society, technology and belief systems.

CHAPTER 9

When Intervention Is Needed

In previous chapters, we focused on lifestyle methods to keep your body and mind vibrant for as long a period as possible. You have learned how to age at a half the rate as your peers who live a typical lifestyle.

However, ultimately we may require intervention, i.e., external help. There are many interventional methods, synthetic drugs, open surgeries, stem cells, gene therapies, hormone replacement therapies and minimally invasive surgeries, just to name a few.

In this chapter, we'll survey a few effective interventional methods, which are still in the category of "natural," rather than "chemical" or "synthetic" or "invasive" which we believe have huge potential in extending our productive years. Lifestyle combined with these "natural" interventional methods will form the basis of a new medicine.

It's important that you work to extend your youthful vitality for as long as possible using lifestyle methods covered in Chapters 1–8, before interventional methods may become necessary.

9.1   THE NEW MEDICINE

Mankind is facing the major challenge of supporting a large increase in the aging population and the resulting increase of all the degenerative diseases such as cancer, Alzheimer's, diabetes, cardiovascular disease, Parkinson's, osteoporosis, macular degeneration, arthritis and many others.

"Over the course of the next 25 years, the age structure of the world population will continue to shift, with older age groups making up an increasingly larger share of the total. For example, during the 1998–2025 period, the world's elderly population (ages 65 and above) will more than double while the world's youth (population under age 15) will grow by 6 percent, and the number of children under age 5 will increase by less than 5 percent. As a result, world population will become progressively older during the coming decades.

Because of population aging, old age dependency ratios will rise in every major world region during the next 25 years. And the world community as a whole will face an elderly support burden nearly 50 percent larger in 2025 than in 1998."

—U.S. CENSUS BUREAU

Medical care cost is at the center of heated discussion in almost every country and is the subject of extensive media coverage. It has become clear: Simply employing conventional medicine to deal with the future elderly population, the cost will become prohibitive for any country to shoulder.

We submit that a new medicine, and shift of paradigm, must be the future of medical treatment. The new medicine will, in combination of the continued conventional advancement, dramatically lower the total medical cost and become the breakthrough solution to mankind in resolving one of the greatest challenges of the coming decades.

9.1.1   Advanced Diagnostic Technology for Sub-Health

Apart from the "pass/fail" or "negative/positive" of conventional medicine, the new medicine will routinely be able to detect sub-health conditions far ahead of any developed disease conditions, even long before any symptoms occur. We have already incorporated many state-of-the-art diagnostics in the PingLongevity™ Test presented in Section 1.4.4.

9.1.2   Natural Medicine Is Replacing Synthetic Drugs

The new medicine will be all natural, using highly concentrated, highly bio-available herbal and natural supplements, rather than synthetic drugs. New manufacturing technology has been increasingly enabling the extraction of natural substances with hundreds of times more bioavailability than, for example, Traditional Chinese Medicine preparations.

> "I am a family physician, who has had leaky gut syndrome for more than 10 years, with many intestinal ulcers. It is a very common 'un-treatable' disease. This triggers an autoimmune reaction, which had led to gastrointestinal problems such as abdominal bloating, excessive gas and cramps, fatigue, food sensitivities, joint pain, skin rashes and autoimmunity. Live and dry blood under dark field microscope showed lots of stuff that doesn't belong in normal healthy blood. I've been to specialist after specialist with no result. All they tell me is that I have an autoimmune disorder.
>
> "I was lucky to be referred to Dr. Ping. Through a series of tests, I was found severely deficient in essential amino acids, the building blocks of all of our body systems. The tests further showed that I was not deficient in protease, the enzyme for digesting proteins. Somehow, I was not able to absorb proteins, which may be the reason for the ulcers in my digestive tract. Upon using a very high bio-available protein supplement, within a few weeks, upon another colonoscopy and amino acid test, it was found that my intestine has completely healed and my amino acid levels are back to normal!"
>
> —JENNIFER, LOS ANGELES

9.1.3   Biomedical Technology Is Becoming Mainstream Medicine

Dr. David Ho, a famous American Chinese scientist at the Aaron Diamond AIDS Research Center, in remarks made during the 2010

Global Views Business Forum in Taipei, has predicted that there will be a shift of pharmaceutical and biomedical emphasis from small molecules to large molecules. Indeed, this will a part of the makings of the new medicine.

A small molecule is a low molecular weight organic compound, which is by definition not a biopolymer. Biopolymers include large molecules such as proteins and nucleic acid (e.g., DNA). In the past, billions dollars have been devoted to discovering small molecule synthetic drugs. However, recent advancement in stem cell technology and gene therapy have demonstrated huge promise in treating many degenerative diseases as we will discuss in the following sections.

If you Google the name John Brodie, the famous San Francisco 49ers American football quarterback, you will find the story about his recovery from a massive stroke that left him paralyzed and with speech problems. After years of treatment with no progress, he went through stem cell therapy. Now, he's back to playing golf, has regained his speech and travels the world by himself. This is what this breakthrough biomedical technology promises.

9.1.4   Back to Ancient Holistic Roots

Modern medicine, or conventional Western medicine, born in the 19th century, has made significant breakthroughs in the past 100 years, including the discovery of miracle drugs like penicillin and other antibiotics. However, this view of symptom-based medicine is a dramatic departure from philosophies of the ancient holistic medicines, such as the Traditional Chinese Medicine. The new medicine will bring us back to our holistic roots:

- It will consider the entire body as an interconnected whole. One example is the hormone therapies we discussed in Chapter 7. All the hormonal axes are an interconnected web (Section 7.3). In treatment, we must consider the entire body, all organs and all systems;

- It emphasizes the ancient TCM philosophy taught by Bian Que thousands of years ago, that "Top doctors prevent diseases before they manifest, middle level doctors heal sub-health and bottom level doctors treat diseases." Therefore preventative medicine will be a part of regular treatment;

- It integrates body, mind and spirit, which has been demonstrated throughout this book and PingLongevity™.

9.2 BIO-IDENTICAL HORMONE REPLACEMENT THERAPY

In Chapter 7, we discussed several ways of keeping your hormone levels balanced, including lifestyle, Taoist alchemy, food therapy and natural hormone balancing using herbs and supplements. When all these methods fail to sustain your youthful hormones, more potent methods may be warranted. This involves using real hormones.

There are several primary hormone replacement therapies (HRT). Synthetic hormone replacement, for example, in treating female hormone imbalance, uses drugs such as Premarin™ and Progestin™. These are synthetic patentable hormones that are different in chemical structure from the hormones in the human body. Study after study has demonstrated that this method is unsafe.

It is not clear why these synthetic hormones cause such serious side effects. It may be due to their different molecular structure, or due to the increased potency of the individual hormones, or simply because the wrong treatment protocol was used. As discussed in Section 7.3, it is difficult to individually tailor hormone replacement therapy so that it corrects imbalances and diminished hormone levels.

Bio-identical hormone replacement therapy (BHRT), another class of hormone replacement therapy, refers to the use of hormones that are molecularly identical to the hormones made by your own body. This class of hormones is not patentable and thus not marketed by pharmaceutical companies. However, they are FDA approved and a prescription is required to purchase them. They are individually formulated by compounding pharmacies.

Despite the potential benefit of being molecularly identical to the natural hormones produced in our bodies and the claim by many well-known anti-aging doctors that BHRT is safe and effective in treating many degenerative diseases, unlike synthetic hormones, there have been no large-scale comprehensive studies on their safety and efficacy.

Many professional societies and regulatory agencies, including the International Menopause Society, American Congress of Obstetricians and Gynecologists, United States Food and Drug Administration, American Association of Clinical Endocrinologists, American Medical Association and the American Cancer Society have released statements that the there is a lack of evidence that the benefits and risks of BHRT are different from well-studied non-bioidentical counterparts, that until such evidence is produced, the risks should be treated as if they were similar. These organizations also caution that compounded hormone products may have additional risks related to compounding.

We believe that BHRT should be the choice over synthetic hormone replacement. But BHRT definitely has risk. However, the risk is not in the hormones themselves, it is in the complexity of using them. If we use the wrong hormones, or the wrong dosage, or the wrong combination, sequential order, timing (Section 7.3), or wrong target (Section 7.4.1) or use the wrong testing methods (Section 1.4.1), we may create a negative impact on our total control system, resulting in side effects. Therefore, if you need hormone replacement therapy, make sure to find a doctor who knows how to do it correctly.

With the correct application, BHRT can be a very good interventional method.

9.3   STEM CELL TECHNOLOGIES

In what has been interpreted as an effort to move forward biomedical research, President Obama signed an executive order ending an $8^{1}/_{2}$-year ban on federal funding for embryonic stem cell research, paving the way for a significant amount of federal funds to flow to science.

"Scientists believe these tiny cells may have the potential to help us understand, and possibly cure, some of our most devastating diseases and conditions."
—BARACK OBAMA

On Jan. 21, 2009, just a day after Mr. Obama's inauguration, Geron received FDA clearance to begin the world's first human clinical trial of embryonic stem cell-based therapy for acute spinal cord injury.

Apparently the world powers are competing for breakthroughs in biomedical technologies that will save lives and solve the heavy burden of health care costs on national resources.

There's no doubt that stem cell research has significant potential. Empirically, there have been many clinical cases showing dramatic improvement of disease conditions such as spinal cord injury, stroke, heart disease, cancer, diabetes, Parkinson's, multiple sclerosis, severe burns, ALS, Huntington's, lupus, sickle cell anemia, HIV/AIDS, osteoarthritis, rheumatoid arthritis and vision and hearing loss.

The potential of breakthrough medicine to change lives of millions people and to solve one of the biggest problems of the society is huge, given that:

- There is an epidemic of neurological and cardiovascular diseases on a global scale;

- Blindness affects 30 million Americans, 90 million in 20 years;

- Macular degeneration affects 33% of the U.S. population over 74;

- Alzheimer's disease and senile dementia affect 50% of the American population over age 82;

- Traumatic Brain Injury (TBI)—the leading cause of death/disability for Americans under the age of 45, with 5.3 million are currently disabled from TBI;

- Strokes affect 750,000 Americans each year with 160,000 deaths, 6 million current survivors;

- Parkinson's affects over 1 million in the U.S.

9.3.1   What Is a Stem Cell?

Stem cells are the "master" cells that give rise to each of the specialized cells within your body. They possess the two properties of:

- Self-renewal: the ability to go through numerous cycles of cell division while maintaining the undifferentiated state;

- Potency: the capacity to differentiate into specialized cell types.

During organ and tissue development, stem cells transform into particular specialized cells, such as nerve, muscle, skin, bone, cartilage, blood and organs (brain, pancreas, lung, heart), when prompted by their environment or by genetic programs that live within them. Stem cells also renew themselves while maintaining their transformative potential. It is the body's own renewal and regenerative mechanism!

From the time an egg is fertilized by a sperm, stem cells go through several stages of maturity.

- Omnipotent stem cells generally refer to approximately the first 10 days from conception. Embryonic stem cells give rise to all cell types. In this stage, the egg is fertilized by a single sperm cell and forms a blastocyst;

- The next stage of development is pluripotent stage, in which the stem cells can give rise to all cell types in their germ layer, ectoderm, mesoderm, endoderm;

- In the multipotent stage, which starts approximately three weeks later, stem cells can generate only major cell types of their tissue of origin;

- The last stage is tissue specific stem cells, in which stem cells reside in stem cell niche within the organ.

Depending on their properties, stem cells are classified into multiple types:

- Embryonic stem cells are cultures of cells derived from the epiblast tissue of the inner cell mass (ICM) of a blastocyst or earlier morula stage embryos. Generally they fall within the stages of omnipotent and pluripotent.

- Fetal stem cells are primitive cell types found in the organs of fetuses and generally, refer to fetal cells approximately three weeks after conception and fall within pluripotent and multipotent stages.

- Adult stem cells refers to any cell that is found in a developed organism that has two properties: the ability to divide and create another cell like itself and also divide and create a cell more differentiated than itself. They are lineage-restricted and are generally referred to by their tissue origin (mesenchymal stem cell, adipose-derived stem cell, endothelial stem cell, etc.). They generally belong to the stages of multipotent and tissue specific.

- Induced pluripotent stem cells are a type of stem cells artificially made by genetic reprogramming with protein transcription factors. Many scientists believe that this class of man-made stem cells can be identical to embryonic stem cells.

Adult stem cells reside in blood, fat tissues, bone marrow and organs. They are our body's natural agents for regeneration and repair.

However, as we age, the total number of stem cells is reduced and quality of stem cells is compromised. For example, in bone marrow, the total number of stem cells sharply decreases from an average of 1 in 20,000, to 1 in 2,000,000 bone marrow cells from newborn to age 80! Thus we lose regenerative capability as we age.

Stem cell therapy promises to use stem cells to enhance the body's own regenerative capability to help treat, regenerate and repair our aged or diseased bodies.

9.3.2 Stem Cell Treatment—Risk and Promise

Stem cell treatments can be classified as:

- Autologous stem cells, in which stem cells are harvested from and put back into the patient; and

- Allogeneic stem cells, in which stem cells harvested from a different person are used. In allogeneic treatment, it is further classified as adult allogeneic therapy, which uses adult stem cells and fetal stem cells after approximately 3 weeks of development and embryonic ones, using embryonic stem cells.

The methods of treatment can also be further divided into:

- Stem cells without expansion and banking, in which stem cells are extracted from the donor and put into the patient, without any manipulation (e.g., culturing to make more stem cells) and storage (freezing), usually in an autologous treatment;

- Stem cells without expansion, same as above, except they can be stored for future use, usually in an autologous treatment;

- Stem cell therapy, in which stem cells are harvested from donor tissues, expanded into many more cells, purified, safety checked, stored and administered into the same patient (autologous) or patients (allogeneic).

Since the first two do not involve any stem cell manipulation, they are similar to cell therapy, for example, in blood infusion, dialysis (blood filtering), organ transplant, bone marrow transplant, all involving stem cells in the transplantation, however, without specific stem cell manipulation.

In stem cell treatment, generally there are a number of concerns: safety, potency and efficacy, quality and treatment protocols.

Safety considerations are:

- Autologous vs. allogeneic: Autologous treatment using your own stem cell is safer than allogeneic one using donor cells.

- The amount of manipulation of cells: Usually the less manipulation in the stem cell used in the treatment, the safer it is. Therefore, stem cell transplantation without expansion and banking is the safest. The more manipulation there is, the more potentially unknown factors may be introduced, including processing issues, impurities and shelf life.

- The cell stage used: Generally, the earlier development stage of the stem cell, such as embryonic stem cell, the more technologically challenging it is to control the behavior of the cell in the body. For example, how do you control the stem cells not to replicate themselves into tumor cells? Thus, in general, adult stem cells are safer than embryonic stem cells and induced pluripotent stem cells, because they have limited replications and directions for proliferation into specific type of cells.

By potency, in general, we refer to the ability of stem cells to engraft into the body, migrate to an injury site and differentiate into the expected specific cell types in order to treat specific diseases. Generally, the more potent the stem cells, the more effective they are in disease treatment. Potency is also generally the inverse of safety, namely, the earlier stage, the more potent, the more manipulation, the better results and allogeneic being more effective than autologous. Therefore, the challenge of the sciences is to find potent, yet safe solutions.

The quality of stem cells means a producer can produce cells with high potency and safety, consistently, from batch to batch. When penicillin was first introduced, a large number of people had allergic reactions to the drug. It became necessary to conduct a skin test prior to injection. Nowadays, a skin test is seldom necessary because of consistent high manufacturing quality. In stem cells, it's the same principle. You must know you are using a high quality source.

Stem cell treatment is also a science. For example, where and how do the doctors inject the cells, intravenously or directly at the injury sites (e.g., heart, eyes, spinal cord)? What's the dosage and how often?

Not all stem cells are equal. It's like riding a horse. You may get a donkey mistaken for a horse; you may get a dead horse or a sick and old horse or a wildly unrideable untrainable horse or a fast and strong champion horse. This is where technology in manufacturing, quality control, safety, potency and treatment protocol differentiate.

There are lots of empirical stem cell treatments showing very promising results. They are mostly in the following areas:

- Disease and injury treatment: There are cases of success in treating spinal cord injury, stroke, heart disease, cancer, diabetes, Parkinson's, Alzheimer's, multiple sclerosis, severe burns, ALS, Huntington's disease, lupus, sickle cell anemia, HIV/AIDS, osteoarthritis, rheumatoid arthritis and vision and hearing loss, autism, diabetic retinopathy, macular degeneration, burns and arthritis, just to name a few.

- Anti-aging and sub-health rejuvenation: In people who are in sub-health conditions with symptoms such as lack of energy, lack of sexual vitality, insomnia and pain, stem cell treatment has shown positive results.

- Cosmetics and aesthetics: Stem cells can be directly injected into the face, hands, neck and scars to rejuvenate the skin, help regrow collagen and fat and grow new blood vessels for better circulation to the skin. They can also inserted into fat tissues to enhance the survival rate during fat grafting procedures. Stem cells contain hundreds of growth factors and cytokines. They can be formulated into facial creams for facial rejuvenation. The main growth factors, for example, are: PDGF (derived growth factor platelet), TGF-b (transforming growth factor beta), EGF (epidermal growth factor), VEGF (vascular endothelial growth factor), IGF-I (insulin-like growth factor I) and bFGF (basic fibroblast growth factor). The main cytokines are: interleukins (IL) 1 to 15, interferons (IF): alpha, beta, gamma, tumor necrosis factor (TNF) alpha and beta, colony stimulating factors (CSF), transforming growth factor (TGF) and other growth factors (PDGF).

9.3.3   Ethical Considerations

Stem cell therapy has been widely used in clinical treatment in the past several years, especially outside the United States and the European Union. Despite showing many cases of success in conventionally untreatable diseases, there are indeed many ethical issues. In most cases, there is no clear manufacturing policy and regulation.

GMP, the standard for manufacturing drugs for human use, is inadequate for manufacturing live human stem cells. In many cases, the stem cells are made in small laboratories without proper certification. In addition, there is often a lack of clinical trial standards. This is because stem cell treatment is a brand new frontier of biomedical sciences. Authorities in many countries have yet to possess the capability to monitor safety and efficacy standards, as well as manufacturing standards. Therefore, in seeking stem cell treatment, care must be taken to minimize the risk.

9.4   GENE THERAPY

Gene therapy is another advanced biotechnology that holds great promise for future biomedical breakthroughs. Currently, gene therapy is used for testing hereditary diseases, susceptibility testing for many degenerative diseases and in certain experimental clinical treatments, such as cancer.

Chromosomes containing our genes are found inside the nucleus of each cell in our bodies. A gene reflects our heredity, defined by a stretch of DNA that encodes instructions on how to make protein or RNA chains. Genes hold the information necessary to build and maintain our cells and pass genetic traits to our offspring. Proteins perform most life functions and make up the majority of the body's cellular structures.

Telomeres are short bits of specialized DNA that cap the chromosomes at the tip, acting as a cellular clock. Over time, cells divide continuously to keep the body alive. But with each cell division, the telomeres get shorter. When they become too short, the cell stops dividing and lapses into a state called cell senescence. Vital tissues are no longer produced and organs start to fail.

Sometimes genes do not function properly because there is an error in the genetic code. If a gene has an error, it is said to be mutated or altered, it is called a single nucleotide polymorphism (SNP), pronounced snip. When a gene with a mistake is passed along in families, it is called an inherited altered gene. When a gene is altered, the encoded proteins are unable to carry out their normal functions and genetic disorders may result.

Classical genetic diseases include, for example, Angelman syndrome, Canavan disease, celiac disease, Charcot-Marie-tooth disease, color blindness, cri du chat, cystic fibrosis, Down syndrome, Duchenne muscular dystrophy, hemochromatosis, hemophilia, Klinefelter's syndrome, neurofibromatosis, phenylketonuria, polycystic kidney disease, Prader-Willli syndrome, sickle-cell disease, Tay-Sachs disease, Turner syndrome.

Other diseases—also partially influenced by lifestyle—that can run through family trees are, for example, certain forms of cancer, cardiovascular disease, diabetes and neurological disorders such as Alzheimer's. Some scientists believe that many health problems can be caused at least in part by altered "histone modifications," and their effects on DNA in cells.

> "We believe that many diseases that have aberrant gene expression at their root can be linked to how DNA is packaged and the actions of enzymes such as histone deacetylases, or HDACs."
> —PROF. ROD DASHWOOD, LINUS PAULING INSTITUTE

9.4.1   Gene Activation

Possessing a "bad" gene is not enough to cause a disease. The gene must be activated, or turned on, or expressed.

Our bodies have a mechanism to turn on and off genes because cells in our bodies need to produce specific proteins at different times in their lives, to help them respond and adapt to changes in their environment.

The DNA double strands need to be 'melted out' and separated in order for the genetic code to be accessed. Most of the time, the gene is kept from being activated by RNA polymerase, which uses a tightly regulated internal blocking system. DNA is activated only when RNA polymerase is modified by an activator protein, which the cell sends to the site of the gene that needs to be switched on.

It has been accepted by most scientists that gene expression is affected by both genetics, i.e., the genes you inherited from your parents and environment, i.e., your lifestyle. Although there are no consistent figures, some scientists say, gene expression is determined 30% by genetic and 70% through lifestyle. Research has revealed how environmental influences strongly affect the way the genetic code at conception is "expressed," or activated. The expression of genes can change rapidly over time; they can be influenced by external factors; those changes can in turn be passed along to offspring. They literally hold the keys to life and death.

Take cancer, and perhaps many other diseases, for example. Compounds in food, such as sulforaphane in broccoli, indole-3-carbinol in cruciferous vegetables and organosulfur in garlic and onions, can act as inhibitors, which prevent cancer genes from being activated. Other examples include butyrate, an inhibitor compound produced in the intestine when dietary fiber is fermented. This provides one possible explanation for why higher intake of dietary fiber might help prevent cancer.

> "Metabolism seems to be a key factor, too, generating the active HDAC inhibitor at the site of action. In cancer cells, tumor suppressors such as p21 and p53 often become epigenetically silenced. HDAC inhibitors can help turn them on again, and trick the cancer cell into committing suicide via apoptosis. We already know some of the things people can do to help prevent cancer with certain dietary or lifestyle approaches. Now we're hoping to more fully understand the molecular processes going on, including at the epigenetic level. This should open the door for new approaches to disease prevention or treatment through diet, as well as in complementing conventional drug therapies."
> —PROF. ROD DASHWOOD, LINUS PAULING INSTITUTE

Therefore, your lifestyle can not only dramatically influence your health and longevity, but also influence the wellbeing of your offspring. The lifestyle choices covered in Chapters 1 through 8 are very important. You cannot blame all of your health on genetic pre-destination. Take control of your health and longevity!

9.4.2   Genetic Testing

Gene testing is used to detect genetic diseases, such as celiac disease, and susceptibility to certain common complex conditions, which are not only dependent on genes, but also on lifestyle, such as heart disease, diabetes and cancer.

In gene tests, DNA samples are obtained from blood, saliva, hair or by scraping cells from inside the cheek. The sampled DNA can be compared to the sequence of normal DNA to discover abnormality or mutation.

For most degenerative diseases, genetic testing can only indicate your risk of developing such conditions as heart disease, diabetes, cancer, etc. All these conditions depend also on lifestyle. Therefore, gene testing has a limited use beyond identifying pure genetic diseases.

The other limitation of gene testing is that it can only test a limited number of gene mutations, which are known to us for particular disease conditions. A positive result may not indicate all of the genes involved in the condition.

9.4.3   Gene Therapy

Gene therapy attempts to correct defective genes responsible for diseases. It has been showing promise in some clinics, especially in treating cancers.

The methods are mainly:

- To insert a functional gene to replace a nonfunctional gene in the genome;

- To swap an abnormal gene for a normal one through homologous recombination;

- To repair a faulty gene through selective reverse mutation

- To turn on or off a particular gene.

Gene therapy no doubt will provide breakthrough therapies in the future.

9.5 ORGAN REPLACEMENT

Organ replacement, or even more generally, body part replacement, makes it possible to dramatically improve the quality of life of many people who otherwise would have been handicapped. The field of organ replacement provides many intervention options.

Advances in prosthetic devices, artificial device extension that replaces a missing body part, have made possible for many life extending procedures, some as simple as dentures to far greater advances, for example joint replacement, prosthetics, artificial heart valves, artificial hearts and lungs, artificial eyes and palatal obturators for cleft palate.

Synthetic vascular grafts make it possible for replacement of whole segments of larger arteries such as the aorta and for use as sewing cuffs.

Advancements in tissue engineering and artificial organs have produced many exciting replacement options such as autologous heart valves and vessels, muscle tissues cultured in vitro, bioartificial liver devices; artificial pancreas, bladders, cartilage, skin, bone marrow and limbs; brain pacemakers and penile, cochlear, retinal and optic nerve implants.

> "Various new technologies, including stem cells, tissue engineering, xenotransplantation and organogenesis, all have potential for replacing or augmenting organ function,"
> —DR. JEFFREY L. PLATT, MAYO CLINIC

Organogenesis involves the growing of a complex organ from primitive cells such as stem cells. For example, led by Dr. Hans Kierstead, researchers at the University of California Irvine have recently announced the successful creation of the world's first human retina made of human embryonic stem cells.

9.6   MINIMALLY INVASIVE SURGERIES

Advancements in medical technologies have enabled an increasingly wide application of non-invasive and minimally invasive surgeries to address many disease related to aging.

Non-invasive surgeries referred to any procedure that does not require direct penetration of the skin. It is usually performed by lasers. For example, lasers are used to shrink tumors, remove moles, warts and other skin blemishes. They are used to remove hair and reduce wrinkles in the skin. Lasik eye surgery is another form of non-invasive surgery that uses a laser to reshape the cornea to correct vision problems.

Of special interest here is a class of minimally invasive surgeries where the incision is so small that no stitches are needed. A classic example is laparoscopic surgery, a type of surgery that is performed with the use of keyhole incisions guided by a light and camera, a scope and sometimes robots, allowing a surgeon to work without creating a large incision.

For example, Dr. David Ditsworth of the Spine Institute pioneered the non-dramatic spine surgery that uses a small endoscope with an incision less than 0.16 inches (4mm) long, inserted from the side of the waist through fascia to correct disc issues without touching bones, muscles and nerves.

The technique is also used in heart surgeries, avoiding open surgeries that require an external artificial heart pump.

Cancer treatment is another area of increased application. Nowadays, many forms of tumor can be removed without open surgeries, for example, brain, lung, sinus and liver cancers.

Another application is interventional radiology, which delivers chemotherapy directly to the affected organ, killing the tumor with heat or freezing the tumor to treat cancer locally, without harming the healthy cells in the body. Success has been demonstrated in treatment of liver cancer, bone tumors, renal tumors, kidney cancer and lung cancer.

9.7 TINKERING WITH THE CLOCK

Our internal cellular clock is measured by telomeres, structures at the very tip of each arm of the chromosome (Section 9.4). A telomere has a length measured in microscopic units called "bases." At conception, these telomeres are approximately 15,000 bases long. Immediately after conception, cells begin to divide and telomeres begin to shorten each time the cell divides. Once your telomeres have been reduced to about 5,000 bases, you essentially die of old age. Thus cell division is limited to 75–100, i.e., the so-called Hayflick Limit.

Reproductive cells do not die. They do not undergo the same telomere shortening process as all other cells in your body do. This is due to the presence and production of an enzyme called telomerase. Other cells do also contain genes for telomerase production, however, the gene is turned off.

A 2009 study published in the *Proceedings of National Academy of Sciences*, which focused on Ashkenazi Jews, finds those who lived the longest had inherited a hyperactive version of an enzyme called telomerase that rebuilds telomeres.

> "Our findings suggest that telomere length and variants of telomerase genes combine to help people live very long lives, perhaps by protecting them from the diseases of old age. We're now trying to understand the mechanism by which these genetic variants of telomerase maintain telomere length in centenarians. Ultimately, it may be possible to develop drugs that mimic the telomerase that our centenarians have been blessed with."
> —Dr. Yousin Suh, Yeshiva University

Many scientists are conducting research to find out how to turn the telomerase gene back on in non-reproductive cells. They're doing this by searching for chemical compounds that will bind to the repressor protein, which will allow the gene to turn back on. In the next few years, there will be many synthetic and natural compounds to be discovered to have telomere-altering properties.

For example, in 1999, a University of Wisconsin team, led by Professors Tomas A. Prolla and Richard Weindruch, profiled the actions of 6,347 genes, with respect to changes in genetic activity in two groups of mice, one group on a standard diet and another group whose diet had been reduced to 76% of the standard diet. In 2003, researchers led by Dr. David Sinclair at Harvard Medical School discovered that the gene, PNC1, is required for the lifespan extension that yeast organisms experience under caloric restriction. A yeast strain with five copies of PNC1 lives 70% longer than the wild type strain, the longest lifespan extension yet reported in that organism.

Based on genetic research on caloric restriction, the only scientifically proven way of extending maximum lifespan (Chapter 3), many substances that have a similar impact on genes as caloric restriction, for example, resveratrol, metformin, lipoic acid, 2-deoxy-D-glucose, pterostilbene, quercetin and grape seed polyphenols.

Lifestyle can have a profound impact on the length of telomeres. Studies have shown that athletes had longer telomeres than sedentary individuals. Being obese, lacking omega-3 fatty acids and certain vitamins also shortened the length of telomeres. Stress also reduces the length of telomeres. People who are pessimists have shorter telomeres.

In other studies in caloric restriction, a worm study shows that the two genes which control dauer stage (a kind of hibernation state when there is a lack of food, or overpopulation and the worm enters a state that the metabolic rate is almost zero). When these genes are slightly altered to make a "weak mutation," the worm can double its life span while still living actively and reproducing. This alteration also doubles the worm's youthful lifespan. Some research hypothesized that in humans, the two similar hormones that control our "age clock" are IGF-1 and insulin.

Both IGF-1 and insulin bind on the same type of receptors. The higher the resting insulin rate, the more signals are sent to the aging clock and the faster you age. Therefore, all of us should monitor the trend of this ratio through annual physicals. If the ratio changes over time, measures should be taken to bring it back to balance as soon as possible.

Although we are very early in the discovery stage, the research in telomerase activation and in caloric restriction mimetics are both promising areas to watch.

9.8 SUMMARY

We have surveyed in this chapter various methods of hormone intervention. We summarize the major points below:

- Although the chapter is about interventional methods, we want to remind you that the goal is to use lifestyle methods as discussed in Chapters 1 through 8 to maintain optimal health for as long as you can so you can delay the need for interventional methods as long as possible. There is no "free" one-pill-fits-all elixir for longevity. All interventional methods have some inherent and sometimes unknown risks and potential side effects. What we tried to outline in this chapter are the interventional methods that are more natural and may be less toxic.

- When lifestyle cannot sustain a youthful hormone balance, you should consider bio-identical hormone replacement therapy. Care must be taken to minimize the risk by having a professional who really knows the subject and has a proven track record.

- Stem cell technologies have the potential to become a breakthrough of this era. They have potential not only for effective solutions to many of the degenerative diseases that otherwise have no treatments, but also provide a preventative maintenance, anti-aging, sub-health rejuvenation solution.

- Gene therapy, although unproven, holds huge promise in the future.

- Organ replacement makes it possible to dramatically extend our productive lives instead of becoming handicapped.

- Minimally invasive surgeries will be the surgeries of the future.

- Tinkering with our age clocks, the telomeres, is an exciting area of research. Although it's hard to imagine we can achieve immortality through this, it's possible to dramatically increase healthy maximum lifespan in the future.

Finally, to motivate you do the "hard work" of using lifestyle approaches and delay the need for intervention, let us quote a landmark study to end this chapter.

In 2008, researchers studied a group of men with prostate cancers. Led by Drs. Dean Ornish, Peter Carroll and Christopher Haqq at the University of California, San Francisco, patients were put on a three-month low-fat, plant-based, whole-foods (minimally processed or refined foods such as whole grains) diet. The result was dramatic. More than 500 genes changed the way they worked. Genes with beneficial effects, including some tumor-suppression genes, became more active. Genes with deleterious effects, including some cancer-promoting genes, were switched off.

> "It is absolutely intriguing this lifestyle change can have as much effect as the most powerful drugs available to us now. We medical oncologists are always looking for drugs that can do this. It is delightful to find that diet and lifestyle can have profound effects and work as well as drug therapies with fewer side effects."
>
> —DR. CHRISTOPHER HAQQ, UCSF

CHAPTER 10

Life as Energy

The advancement of science, technology and civilization has been preceded by many people with bold imaginations, hypotheses and dreams, sprinkled with more than a little science fiction. In the life sciences, there are so many unanswered questions. For example, exactly what is "chi," "life force" or "life energy?" What happens when you die? Is there a spirit? Is there afterlife? Is there immortality?

In this chapter, we talk about hypotheses, rather than proven sciences. These theories must be a part of the new medicine because it is essential to integrate mind and spirit to achieve health and longevity.

The 5,000 years of Taoist teachings, combined with results from modern science form the basis of our hypothesis in this chapter.

10.1 THE UNIFIED ENERGY HYPOTHESIS

Five thousand years ago, the Taoist sages of China formulated their philosophy of the universe, the Oracle of Changes (I Ching) and the complex acupuncture meridians as the paths of energy through the human body.

It is remarkable that today's science and technology have confirmed the validity of these ancient perceptions of the world and the human body. It has been found that the meridians of the ancients correspond to paths in the body with low electrical resistance, even though the meridians are not found in modern physiology to correspond to any physical structures, i.e., blood vessels, lymph nodes or nerves.

More amazingly, around 1969, Drs. Gunther Stent, Martin Schonberger, Marie-Louise von Franz and others independently found that the 64 I Ching hexagrams are identical to the genetic code of DNA, which describes the entire living world. This was discovered less than 50 years ago.

How could these ancients be right on the mark? How were they able to perceive truths that even now modern men struggle to measure and comprehend? It's quite a feat for a prehistoric people who had no written language, no science, no technological instruments, no mathematics. They recorded numbers by tying knots in a blade of grass.

The answer, most likely, is that the ancients were a pure and simple people, their observations not obstructed by the hundreds of distractions we have today. They studied existence as it is—a skill now lost, perhaps through evolution. They perceived nature through a clear lens. Stories talk about ancient herbalists discovering many of the precious herbs with powerful medicinal value. It is said that while climbing high in the mountains, they would pass by a new plant and feel a sensation through different body parts. This gave them an understanding of the healing effect of herbs on specific parts of the body.

The ancient Chinese believed that the universe is filled with energy, that energy is everything. Indeed, much of this has been proven: electromagnetic fields, light beams and gravity fields have all been measured. But the ancients, right in so many things, believed in a continuum of energies, from the lowest level (unstable, impure, mortal, coarse, of the lower spectrum) to the highest level (subtle, immortal, infinite, pure, absolute, perfect, refined, of the higher spectrum).

Perfect energy is called the Tao or chi, a force flowing within us and filling the universe. This energy is the perfect combination and balance of yin and yang energy. Once it is divided into yin and yang energy, it gives birth to all forms. Anything with form has limited energy, such as mountains, trees, animals, humans and stones. They have limited energy potential, thus are mortal. As the energy is expended, the energy of the thing with form returns to the universe. The higher the quality of the energy and the slower the consumption rate, the longer the thing stays stable.

Albert Einstein's theory of relativity holds that all energy and matter are interchangeable and that they depend on the speed at which matter is moving or vibrating. As the speed approaches that of light, the energy increases towards infinity and matter becomes mass-less. This is described in Einstein's celebrated mass-energy formula, the Einstein-Lorentz transformation:

$$E \; = \; M \; \frac{c^2}{\sqrt{1 - (v/c)^2}}$$

where E stands for energy, M for mass, c for the speed of light and v for the speed of the mass.

This is in agreement with the ancients who knew the universe is filled with energies. Energies have their associated speed. At lower speeds, energies are condensed into physical existence. As the speed increases, energies become subtle, formless and mass-less. In living things, the higher the vibration of energy, the longer and more stable its life.

Physicists use the term *entropy* to describe the disorganization of things or the randomness of a system. The greater the degree of disorder, the higher is the entropy. In thermodynamics, a formula $S = H - G$ is used to describe the relationship among entropy S, heat H and energy potential available for useful work G in a closed thermodynamic system. Thus, the less the energy potential G, the higher is the entropy S (the tendency toward disorganization). The higher the energy consumed, represented by heat H, the higher is the entropy. Thermodynamics holds that all closed systems (approximately applied to humans, not entirely a closed system) have positive entropy, which always increases as time goes by, so the system ultimately becomes more and more disorganized until it destroys itself and dies. This agrees very much with the ancient Chinese view of the universe that lower energy forms are mortal and unstable.

Until recently, it was considered impossible that energy could vibrate faster than the speed of light. However, physicists have now hypothesized the possibility of a negative space/time. As noted in Einstein's formula, when v is larger than c, energy E becomes an imaginary number, thus the name negative space/time. In such a space/time, energy vibrating faster than the speed of light would cause living systems to possess negative entropy (sometimes called extropy), increasing order and organization as time goes by and actually enhance the system's ability to live a longer, more stable and even immortal existence. The higher the vibration of the energies, the more stable they stay. This hypothesis by modern physicists again agrees with the ancients—the higher the energy, the more immortal it is.

Thus our hypothesis of universal energy suggests that *all things in the universe are energy. The expression of energy forms a continuum depending on vibration speed, from form to formless, from mortal to immortal.*

10.2 THE LIFE ENERGY HYPOTHESIS

The I Ching, when put in the context of life cycle, states that when there is birth, there must be a death. Birth grows out of death, and death occurs in birth. The universe of transformation is periodic and yin-yang balanced.

I Ching represents yin with a broken line and yang with a solid line. Then I Ching stacks six broken and solid lines into a hexagram representing one state. There are 64 different combinations of the six lines, with broken or solid lines in all six positions. These 64 hexagrams represent 64 different states of change in the universe. The hexagram grows from bottom to top. Thus, one broken line at the bottom and five solid lines at the top means there is a recent birth of yin into the new state. When the different hexagrams are put in order, they describe a change process or law in the universe, living things, or events going from one state to another. Life cycle can be expressed as in the diagram on the following page.

Life starts at birth, which is at the full yin state (six yin lines), and

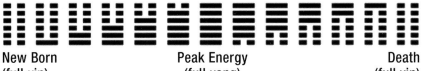

New Born
(full yin)

Peak Energy
(full yang)

Death
(full yin)

reaches its peak energy at full yang state (six yang lines), with a gradual increase of yang from the bottom up, representing the increase of energy. After the peak energy state, life begins a gradual slide. This downhill process is represented by an increase of yin (broken lines) from the bottom up until full yin is reached, when death returns to birth and a cycle ends.

As you can see, if you add the hexagrams together, it is yin-yang balanced (the number of yin and yang are equal, and the periodical life process itself is yin and yang balanced).

"Peak energy" in people occurs at puberty when male and female become capable of reproduction, typified by the first leakage of semen (male) and blood in menstruation (female).

All humans possess three major bands of energies: spirit, chi and essence or physical body. They are energies in three different manifestations with different vibrational speeds, spirit being the highest and essence the lowest. And all humans have pure and impure energy components; the purer they are, the longer they live. Conversely, the more impure they are, the shorter their lives. The faster they consume the limited energy potential, the quicker the rate they travel toward death.

At conception, pure spirit energy enters to combine with the vital essence of the parents (the sperm of the father and egg of the mother) as well as the mother's nursing chi to form the seed of new life. This is the basic beginning of life, the prenatal energy. Inside the womb, yin (in the form of essence) and yang (in the form of spirit) are in perfect union.

At birth, yin and yang separate and the I Ching life cycle begins. Spirit (subconscious mind) and mind (conscious mind) move upward to be housed in the brain and the heart and essence moves down to be stored in the kidneys. Postnatal essence builds up through the digestion of nutrients from food. Together, spirit energy and essence sustain the life force, the chi. Life is supported by chi; strong spirit and essence support strong chi, which in turn supports life. Throughout life, spirit leaks upwards through emotions, while essence leaks downward in the form of enzymes, semen, blood, eggs, body fluids and through the metabolic processes. As vital essence and spirit energies are depleted, chi is gradually weakened. Since chi cannot sustain life, life ends.

Prior to puberty, children are naïve and relatively mindless. They usually do not relate to things like fame, wealth, success, social standards and stress. Therefore, spiritual energy is largely preserved. Leakage of semen in men and blood in women has not begun. Essence is also preserved. Therefore, the life force, or chi energy, is increasing and will peak at puberty.

After puberty, on the spiritual level, stress begins to accumulate. We start to understand power, social status, fame, money, politics, sexual attraction and the pressures of work. The spirit becomes overpowered by modern realities and spirit energy decreases as these take their toll. As spirit energy diminishes, chi is weakened and so, too, is life.

Thus, the hypothesis of life energy assumes that *longevity not only depends on the rate of living (metabolism), i.e., how fast one's limited energy potential is consumed, but also depends on the quality, measured by the vibrational speed based on the hypothesis of universal energy, of one's energy. Furthermore, there's a part of your energy, spiritual energy that is immortal. Through lifelong alchemy, it is possible to increase such immortal energy, making your afterlife stronger.*

10.3 MAXIMUM LIFESPAN

Both the ancient Chinese masters and modern scientists estimate that humans have a maximum life span of 100 to 120 years. In fact, if we could cure all heart disease and all cancer and eliminate all the causes of death written on death certificates today so that all people die only from "natural causes," almost everyone would live to be over 100 years old, according to statistics. Can we have an effective program to help people live to their maximum lifespan of around

100 to 120? Can we dramatically increase this maximum limit to over 200? The answer to both questions is yes. As demonstrated in Chapter 3, people are capable of living much longer than 120 years and doing it in a completely productive manner.

Increasing lifespan and maximum lifespan requires us to make some fundamental changes: To become beings with a higher vibrating energy. As discussed earlier, the stability, longevity and immortality of a form depends on both the rate of energy consumption and the quality of the energy, i.e., its frequency of vibration. The more the energy is taking physical forms, the less its vibrating frequency. The physical form disappears as the speed approaches the speed of light and beyond, as we have seen earlier in Einstein's formula. Spirit energy is the highest and most refined in our human energy spectrum; vital essence such as blood, semen, enzyme and body fluids are lower and coarser energies. They both sustain chi to support the existence of life. At death, our essence is drained and spirit energy is weakened through lifelong consumption. Chi is insufficient to sustain life. Thus, our physical body dies and our spirit energy reunites with the universe.

If we can daily preserve and lower the expenditure of our spirit and essence energy, we can sustain a strong chi longer and achieve longevity towards the human maximum limit. Furthermore, if we can use our vital essence energy as raw materials and refine it into higher chi and spirit energy, we can challenge the maximum limit and move toward immortality, an energy so refined that it lasts forever.

How do we preserve and refine our energies? We need to prevent unnecessary expenditure of vital essences, such as blood, semen, enzymes and body fluids. We need to open and balance our energy meridians and centers in order not to accumulate illness (caused by imbalance and blockage) and to be in touch with the infinite cosmic energy source of the universe. We need to calm our spirit from all emotional stress to preserve our spirit energy. We need to transmute the essence energy into higher chi and spirit energy.

This is the basis of previous chapters, in which we discussed methods that minimize the rate of energy expenditures through diet, caloric restriction, exercise, alchemy and mind and spiritual energy preservation.

10.4 IMMORTALITY

While no one knows what immortality is, through our hypothesis of unified energy and life energy, we can assume that a piece of us, our spiritual energy, will live and be immortal. There will be a difference among all the spirits in the afterlife because of their energies. Some will be strong, some very weak.

Taoism believes that if we can maximally extend our healthy physical form (the lower energy components), we can buy time to transmute our energies from lower vibrational frequencies to higher ones, thus ultimately becoming higher spiritual beings. Therefore, when we're talking about immortality, we do not mean physical immortality.

The purpose of Taoist alchemy is to refine postnatal essence into spirit energy, thus increasing our spirit energy potential. Through a lifetime of practice, we have the opportunity to dramatically strengthen spirit energy, thus not only sustaining a very long youthful life, but also elevating into higher beings, the immortals. When this happens, the physical body becomes irrelevant. Immortals can switch between physical bodies and subtle energies.

This explanation of immortality is beyond current science and technology. However, there have been observations of such energy transformation. One was reported in the authoritive book *I Ching and Traditional Chinese Medicine* by Dr. Yang Li. During a mission in May 1987, the Russian space shuttle encountered a strong set of "lights." It consisted of seven huge human-like objects with wings and foggy light rings. Appearing to be several hundred feet tall, they followed the shuttle for at least ten minutes and were recorded on video for 43 minutes. The Russian physicist Monagov said, "These things no doubt were some type of human-like beings. However, they have evolved into a stage so advanced that they can transition between physical bodies and a set of light clouds."

This event has raised many questions: Can human beings evolve into an advanced state where they can transition between different times and spaces instantaneously? How do all these different times and spaces relate to each other? After death, does their spirit transition to another time and space to continue to live? Under what conditions can they return to the human physical world? Some scientists postulate that human genetics must be beyond four-dimensional time and space. After all, within seven weeks of growth, an embryo has repeated 300 million years of evolution. This process must be beyond our comprehension of time and space. It must be beyond the speed of light.

After all, we have immortals right with us. Our genes are immortal. They pass from generation to generation.

10.5 ALCHEMY FOR A STRONGER SPIRIT

In Chapters 5 and 6, we introduced a method of Taoist alchemy. It is not only for the preservation of our life force, but more importantly, for transmuting our most potent life force into spiritual energy. Through this transmutation, Taoists believe that we can ultimately achieve a much stronger higher vibrational spiritual energy in order to attain immortality. In essence, the sexual energy becomes the raw materials for the elixir of immortality.

Taoist alchemy started with the first Chinese king, Huang Di (the Yellow Emperor), five millennia ago. Taoist alchemy believes in self-cultivation and refinement. It is a science set out to explain the laws of the universe and life. It is about the macrocosm of the universe and the microcosm of humans. It observes nature to understand human beings and observes human beings to understand the universe. In development and verification over several thousands of years, Taoist alchemy became the science and the art of self-refinement of spiritual (original nature) and physical (vital life force) lives. Its ultimate goal is to combine life with the Tao, or the ultimate universal chi (energy), to achieve longevity. It believes that our limited life force has all it takes to refine ourselves into immortality and grand happiness, regardless of fate. It is up to us to achieve it.

Taoist alchemy believes in the combined training of both spirit and physical body. It appears to be between religion (pure spiritual) and science (pure material). It requires that body, mind and spirit be one and that the macrocosm of the universe and the microcosm of the human be one. It is through this combination that man, with very limited life, can achieve immortality by communicating with the infinite energy of the universe. According to the old Taoist saying, "The universe has a limited life span; my spirit energy can last forever!"

Chi-gong is the best medium to condition our bodies and minds into the spiritual energy space. Once we can connect ourselves to this high level energy plane, we open ourselves to become higher beings, more spiritually developed, able to communicate with the immortal energy source of the universe, able to change between physical and spiritual planes any time we want and ultimately able to become immortal and forever young. We may never get to the ultimate state of energy, but even just 10% of that is quite a reward for those who seek to stay younger longer and live in good health for more years.

Why is chi-gong able to create such miracles? Humans have a much larger innate capacity to live than we usually tap into. When a typical person dies, he or she has used only 20% of the brain cells, 20% of micro blood vessels and 50% of the DNA capacity available. The human body also has incredible metabolism, digestion and heart muscle fiber capacity. This extra capacity can be used through chi-gong.

The human brain has two aspects, consciousness and sub-consciousness. During billions of years of evolution, the subconscious mind is largely suppressed. We are much less intuitive than people were thousands of years ago. There are still people, the psychic ones, who can sense past and future, who help law enforcement search for criminals by their intuition rather than reasoning. Most of them would say they seem connected with a mysterious force or person that gives them signals. Some animals get very restless right before an earthquake. Some of us feel something strange happening when a relative dies or during other big events, happy or unhappy.

Some of us even have dreams about future events. This is the working of the subconscious mind. Chi-gong is meant to explore the remaining 80% of our brain cells. It is believed this part of the brain, although rarely used, contains unawakened information, such as pre-life memories, space and time communication of past and future, sensing signals that most of us cannot perceive. Thus chi-gong can reverse evolution and unleash the vast power of the brain

An interesting experiment was conducted by Dr. Justa Smith, a biochemist. She wondered if laying-on-hands healing could actually affect a body's enzyme system. You will recall that enzymes are the agents that activate all the body biochemical processes, i.e., metabolism. Different enzymes target different processes, such as digestive enzymes for decomposing food. Dr. Smith found that healers can either speed up activity for some types of enzymes or slow down others. Since healers did not know which enzymes govern which activities, the energy or chi that was passed to the enzymes by healers seemed to have some "intelligence," i.e., selectivity. Dr. Smith further studied a biochemistry flowchart to see where each of the "treated" enzymes fit into the normal pathways of cellular energy metabolism. She observed that the change of enzyme activity produced by the healers was always in the direction of greater energy reserve and increased health of the body's cells. Therefore, the healers' energy, or chi, knows exactly which enzymes to accelerate or decelerate.

As we discussed in Sections 10.1 and 10.2, the human system, like other thermodynamic systems, follows the direction of the second law of thermodynamics. It possesses the property of positive entropy, always going from a more organized state to a less organized state. Entropy thus describes the aging process. Dr. Smith's experiments showed that the energy (or chi) imparted by healers possesses properties that reduce entropy because it always moved the system toward a more organized state. Some physicists call this property "negative entropy" or extropy. If a healer treats cancer, the enzymes that promote cancer growth are inhibited, while the enzymes that promote immune response are strengthened automatically. The exact mechanism of the human energy system is patently unclear to modern technology and science at their current level of understanding.

If, through chi-gong, we can achieve negative entropy, which is immortal by definition, our job becomes to use our body's resources during our lifetime to maximize the energy component in us, which possesses negative entropy. If we can do this as much as possible, we are cultivating the most negative entropy component of our total energy and we are closer to true immortality.

To unleash the great power of the brain is to awaken and strengthen the spirit energy. It is similar to the alchemy process in chemistry. It requires raw materials to start with. In Taoist alchemy, sexual energy is the raw material from which greater spirit energy is refined and stored.

10.6 SUMMARY

We attempted in this chapter to elevate our attention toward a much higher objective, namely to become higher spiritually developed beings. In particular, we hypothesized that:

- All things in the universe are energy. The expression of energy forms a continuum depending on vibration speed, from form to formless, from mortal to immortal.

- Longevity not only depends on the rate of living (metabolism), i.e., how fast one's limited energy potential is consumed, but also depends on the quality, measured by the vibrational speed based on the hypothesis of universal energy, of one's energy. Furthermore, there's a part of your energy, spiritual energy, which is immortal. Through lifelong alchemy, it is possible to increase such immortal energy, making your after life stronger and longer.

- Taoism believes that if we can maximally extend our healthy physical form (the lower energy components), we can buy time to transmute our energies from lower vibrational frequencies to higher ones, thus ultimately becoming higher spiritual beings. We must set our goals beyond physical health, to become higher spiritual beings.

Epilogue

In a world overloaded with information, we have attempted to summarize in this book the real solutions that are based on what we have learned, experienced and practiced. We have offered you solutions that can really make a big difference in keeping you healthy, young and vibrant for life.

We cautioned you that there is no magic one-shot injection that fixes it all. Real development in body, mind and spirit requires a complete solution, both in terms of lifestyle and advanced biomedical solutions. At first, the concept of absorbing all ten chapters of this book may seem overwhelming. So how would you feel about attaining 50%, 30% or only 10% of what is required? Practicing even a fraction of PingLongevity™ will no doubt give you tremendous headroom for staying young longer and living healthier.

Our bodies, minds and spirits are adaptive. The cleaner you are in body and spirit, the more you rid yourself of physical and psychic toxins. But it can go in the opposite direction, too. The more toxic you are, the more you crave the same. We have seen our own preference in diet naturally change from junk food to super-clean, super-energized food. We have seen our spirits evolve from desiring an ever-indulging materialism to a more spiritual world. We did not force ourselves. Our bodies and our spirits wanted it. And your body and spirit probably do, too. By choosing the right direction, your body will happily adapt.

Wouldn't it be nice to look and feel 10 to 30 years younger than you actually are? Wouldn't it be nice to be full of youthful energy in your 40s, 50s, 60s and beyond?

It's never too late, even if you already suffering from a degenerative disease. You can reverse it. It's never too early, either. Aging begins at puberty. You can preserve energy and stop aging.

Our journey started decades ago when we first opened Ping-Clinic, and the results were first summarized in our book *Ping-Longevity,* and subsequent book *Asian Longevity Secrets.* This volume is more complete. We are sure that the advancement of new biomedical technologies and our own research and development will continue to add new dimensions to our understanding of the aging process, leading to further results.

We invite you to start the journey now. By joining us to make mankind healthier and more spiritually developed, we will all benefit.

Dr. Taichi Tzu
Dr. Ping Wu

References

Chapter 1

Hayflick, Leonard, *How and Why We Age* (Ballantine Books, 1996).

Williams, J.E., *Prolonging Health* (Hampton Roads, 2003).

Wu, Ping Wu and Tzu, Taichi, *Asian Longevity Secrets* (PingClinic Publishing, 2003).

Tzu, Taichi and Wu, Ping, *PingLongevity* (PingClinic Publishing, 2001).

Henig, Robin Marantz, *How a Woman Ages* (Ballantine Books, 1985).

Appleton, Nancy, *Rethinking Pasteur's Germ Theory* (Frog, Ltd., 2002).

Chapter 2

Weaver KL, et al, "The Content of Favorable and Unfavorable Polyunsaturated Fatty Acids Found in Commonly Eaten Fish," *Journal of American Diet Association*, 2008, July, 108(7); 1178–85.

Elias & Dykeman, *Edible Wild Plants* (Sterling Publishing, 1990).

McConnaughey, Evelyn, *Sea Vegetables* (Naturegraph Publishers, 1985).

Stamets, Paul, *Psilocybin Mushrooms of the World* (Ten Speed Press, 1996).

Howell, Edward, *Food Enzymes for Health & Longevity* (Lotus Press, 1994).

Sears, Barry, *The Zone* (Regan Books, 1995).

Milchovich, Sue and Dunn-Long, Barbara, *Diabetes Mellitus*,(Bull Publishing, 1999).

Howell, Edward, *Enzyme Nutrition* (Avery Publishing Group, 1985).

Brand-Miller, Jennie et al, *The Glucose Revolution* (Marlowe & Company, 1999).

Campbell, T. Colin and Campbell Thomas II, *The China Study* (Benbella Books, 2004).

Chen, M. et al, "The Role of Dietary Carbohydrate in the Decreased Glucose Tolerance of the Elderly," *Journal of American Geriatrics*, 1987.

Whang, Sang, *Reverse Aging*, 2004

MacWilliam, Lyle, *Comparative Guide to Nutritional Supplements*, (Northern Dimensions Publishing, 2003).

Lee, Lia and Turner, Lisa, *The Enzyme Cure* (Future Medicine Publishing, 1998).

Chapter 3

Walford, Roy, *The 120 Years Diet* (Four Walls Eight Windows, 2000).

Werner, Michael and Stockli, Thomas, *Life from Light* (Clairview Books, 2007).

Walford, Roy and Lisa, *The Anti-Aging Plan* (Four Wall Eight Windows, 1994).

Chapter 4

Chang, Stephen, *The Book of Internal Exercises* (Strawberry Hill Press) 1978.

Chapter 5

Yanchi, Liu, *The Essential Book of Traditional Chinese Medicine* (Columbia University Press, 1995).

Ni,Maoshing, *The Yellow Emperor's Classic of Medicine* (Shambhala, 1995).

Reid, Daniel, *Chinese Herbal Medicine* (Shambhala, 1993).

Hsu, Hong-yen and Peacher, William (Edited by), *Wellspring of Chinese Medicine, Chang Chung-Ching* (Keats Publishing, 1981).

Lo, Shui Yin, *The Biophysics Basis for Acupuncture and Health* (Dragon Eye Press, 2004).

Chapter 6

Sarno, John, *The Mindbody Prescription* (Warner Books, 1998).

Tsu, Lao, translated by Feng, Gia-Fu and English, Jane, *Tao Te Ching* (Vintage Books, 1972).

Wing, R.L., *The Illustrated I Ching* (Doubleday, 1982).

Becker, Robert *Cross Currents* (Tarcher/Putnam, 1990).

Lau, Kwan, *Feng Shui for Today* (Tengu Books, 1997).

I-Ming, Liu, translated by Cleary, Thomas, *Awakening to the Tao* (Shambhala, 1988).

Nan, Huai-Chin, translated by Chu, Wen Kuan, *Tao & Longevity* (Samuel Weiser, 1984).

Chopra, Depak, *Quantum Healing* (Bantam Books, 1990).

Pert, Candace, *Molecules of Emotion* (Touchstone, 1999).

Wong, Eva (translated by), *Cultivating Stillness* (Shambhala, 1992).

Wong, Eva (translated by), *Teachings of the Tao* (Shambhala, 1997).

O'Leary, A. (1990). Stress, emotion, and human immune function. *Psychological Bulletin, 108*, 363–382.

Chapter 7

Percival, Mark, "Phytonutrients & Detoxificaion," *Clinical Nutrition Insights,* NUT040 1/97 Vol. 5, No. 2.

Zeligs, Michael A., "Diet and Estrogen Status: The Cruciferous Connection," *Journal of Medicinal Food,* Volume 1, Number 2, 1998.

Kensler, Thomas W. et al, "Effects of Glucosinolate-Rich Broccoli Sprouts on Urinary Level of Aflatoxin-DNA Adducts and Phenanthrene Tetraols in a Randomized Clinical Trial in He Zuo Township, Qidong, People's Republic of China," *Cancer Epidemiol Biomarkers Prevention,* 14(11), November 2005.

Brooks, James D. et al, "Potent Induction of Phase 2 Enzymes in Human Prostate Cells by Sulforaphane," *Cancer Epidemiology Biomarkers & Prevention*, Vlo. 10, 949–954, September 2001.

Fahey, J.W. and Talalay, P, "Antioxidant Functions of Sultoraphane: a Potent Inducer of Phase II Detoxication Enzymes," *Food and Chemical Toxicology* 27 (1999) 973–979.

Lord, Richard S. et al, "Estrogen Metabolism and the Diet-Cancer Connection: Rationale for Assessing the Ratio of Urinary Hydroxylated Estrogen Metabolites," *Alternative Medicine Review*, Volume 7, Number 2, 2002.

Styne, Dennis, *Pediatric Endocrinology* (Lippincott Willams & Wilkins, 2004).

Wong, Eva (translated by), *Harmonizing Yin and Yang* (Shambhala, 1997).

Smith, Pamela, *HRT: The Answer* (Healthy Living Books, 2003).

Klatz, Ronald, *Grow Young with HGH* (HarperCollins Publishers, 1997).

Luk, Charles (translated by), *Taoist Yoga* (Samuel Weiser, 1973).

Morgantaler, Abraham, *Testosterone for Life* (McGraw Hill, 2009).

Somers, Suzanne, *Breakthrough* (Crown Publishers, 2008)

Gordon, Mark, *The Clinical Application of Interventional Endocrinology* (Phoenix Books, 2007).

Morley, John Morley and van den Berg, Lucretia, *Endocrinology of Aging* (Humana Press, 2000).

Beiss, Uzzi, *Natural Hormone Balance for Women* (Pocket Books, 2001).

Shippen, Eugene and Fryeer, William, *Testosterone Syndrome* (M. Evans and Company, 1998).

Somers Suzanne, *The Sexy Years* (Crown Publishers, 2004).

Weindruch, Richard and Walford, Roy, *The Retardation of Aging and Disease by Dietary Restriction* (Charles C. Thomas Publisher, 1988).

Chia, Mantak, *Iron Shirt Chi Kung I* (Healing Tao Books, 1986).

Chia, Mantak Chia and Chia, Maneewan, *Fusion of the Five Elements I* (Healing Tao Books, 1997).

Chia, Mantak and Chia, Maneewan, *Bone Marrow Nei Kung* (Healing Tao, 1988).

Chia, Mantak, *Awaken Healing Energy through the Tao* (Aurora Press, 1983).

Chia, Mantak and Wynn, Michael, Taoist *Secrets of Love—Cultivating Male Sexual Energy* (Aurora Press, 1984).

Chang, Stephen, *The Tao of Sexology* (Tao Publishing, 1986).

Leifke, Eckhard et al, "Age-related changes of serum sex hormones, insulin-like growth factor-1 and sex-hormone binding globulin levels in men: cross-sectional data from a healthy male cohort" *Clinical Endocrinology*, Volume 53, Issue 6, pages 689–695, December 2000.

Carruthers, Malcolm, *Androgen Deficiency in the Adult Male* (Informa Healthcare, 2010).

Cleary,Thomas (translated by), *The Secret of the Golden Flower* (Harper SanFrancisco, 1991).

Luk, Charles, *The Secrets of Chinese Meditation* (Samuel Weiser, 1964).

Cleary, Thomas (translated by), *Immortal Sisters* (North Atlantic Books, 1996).

Reid, Daniel, *The Tao of Health, Sex, & Longevity,* (Fireside Books, 1989).

Chenyang, Tian, *China Taoism: Cultivation and Practice of the Life* (Religion Culture Press, 1999).

Chengyang, Tian Chengyang, *Immortality Theory* (Religion Culture Press, 1999).

Chengyang, Tian, *Entrance into Tao* (Religion Culture Press, 1999).

Yang, Liu Hua, translated by Eva Wong, *Cultivating Energy of Life* (Shambhala, 1998).

Dabbs, J/M., "Age and Seasonal Variation in Serum Testosterone Concentration among Men," *Chronobiol Int* 1990; 7:245–9.

Chapter 8

Perricone, Nicholas, *The Wrinkle Cure* (Rodale Books, 2000).

Leffell, David, *Total Skin,* (Hyperion, 2000).

Kobren, Spencer David, *The Bald Truth* (Pocket Books, 1998).

Chapter 9

Hamer, Dean Hamer and Copeland, Peter, *Living with Our Genes* (Anchor Books, 1998).

Gupta, Sanjay, *Cheating Death, The Doctors and Medical Miracles that Are Saving Lives Against All Odds,*(Wellness Central, 2009).

Ridley, Matt, *Genome* (HarperCollins Books, 2000).

Shvarta, Esar, *Biogravics* (Pine Island Press, 1997).

Chapter 10

Davies, Paul, *God & the New Physics* (Touchstone Books, 1984).

Fossel, Michael, *Reversing Human Aging* (William Morrow and Company, 1996).

Hua-Ching, Ni, *The Taoist Inner View of the Universe and the Immortal Realm* (Seven Star Communications, 1996).

Hua-Ching, Ni Hua-Ching, *The Subtle Universal Law and the Integral Way of Life* (Seven Star Communications, 1998).

Li, Yang, *I Ching and Traditional Chinese Medicine,* Beijing Sciences and Technology Press, 1997.

Gerber, Richard, *Vibrational Medicine* (Bear & Company, 2001).

Eckman, Peter, *In the Footsteps of the Yellow Emperor* (Cypress Book Co., 1996).

Wong, Eva, *Taoism* (Shambhala, 1997).

Capra, Fritjof, *The Tao of Physics* (Shambhala, 1991).

Kukav, Gary, *The Dancing Wu Li Masters* (Quill William Morow, 1979).

Kaku, Michio and Thompson, Jennifer, *Beyond Einstein* (Anchor Books, 1995).

Schonberger, Martin, *The I Ching and the Genetic Code* (Aurora Press, 1992).

Index

About the Authors

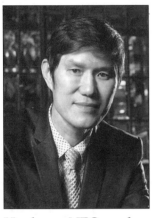

Taichi Tzu, Ph.D., also known as Shu Li, is the chairman of WA Regenerative Medicine Ltd. He is a co-founder of Laguna Beach-based integrative medicine clinic, PingClinic. He is also the holder of the U.S. patent for *Negative Gravity Therapeutic Methods*, and a co-author of the books *PingLongevity* and *Asian Longevity Secrets*. Previously, Dr. Li served as founder, president and CEO of Jazz Semiconductor, as a member of the board of directors of Huahong NEC, and a member of the advisory board at the Paul Merage School of Business Administration, the University of California, Irvine. He also served as senior vice president at Conexant Systems, vice president at AlliedSignal/Honeywell, as well as senior management positions at Motorola and Intel. Dr. Li was on the faculty of the University of Arizona and a partner with the father of Toyota system, Dr. Shigeo Shingo. Dr. Li has published extensively in prestigious scientific journals. He received his Ph.D. in Applied Sciences from Harvard University.

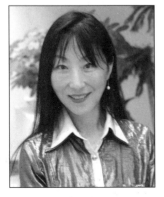

Ping Wu, M.D., Ph.D., O.M.D., M.S., L.Ac. (CA, NCCA), is the founder and Medical Director of the Laguna Beach based integrative medicine clinic, PingClinic. She is the co-author of the books *PingLongevity* and *Asian Longevity Secrets*. Dr. Ping Wu was a recipient of research grants from the American Cancer Society, the University of Arizona Cancer Center and the National Institutes of Health.